D0932683

A BIG HEART

A Memoir

MIKE PAPALE

A BIG HEART

A story about turning trauma into triumph

MIKE PAPALE

A Big Heart is a work of nonfiction.
Copyright © 2021 by Mike Papale
All Rights Reserved

This book or any portion thereof may not be reproduced or used in any
manner whatsoever without the express written permission of the
publisher.
Cover design by Natalie Leroux

To Mom, Dad and John:
I have said from the beginning, it is always harder on the family than it is on the patient. Thank you for all of your love and support.

Foreword

"To save one life is to save the world"

- The Talmud

I had the honor of first meeting Mike Papale in the winter of 2006—our lives colliding in a small sterile examination room in the outpatient cardiology clinic at Tufts Medical Center in Boston. Only a few months earlier, Mike had miraculously survived a near-death event. Like so many survivors of sudden cardiac death, Mike did not know that for the first 17 years of his life, he had actually been living with a heart disease called hypertrophic cardiomyopathy (HCM), which put him at risk—at any moment—of experiencing a life threatening irregular heart rhythm. That all changed on August 24, 2006, when, in the time it took to complete one dribble of a basketball, Mike's heart stopped beating and he came nearer to death than anyone would ever wish to. With the quick and heroic actions of those around him, Mike's heart rhythm was converted to normal and life restored.

The fact that Mike survived this out-of-the-blue, life-threatening cardiac event is itself a miracle. The events of that day are so incredible that one could easily conclude a higher power was looking out for him. And yet, equally amazing is what happened next. What follows here is that story...one that is filled with courage, persistence, strength and the unstoppable passion to prevent sudden cardiac death. As Mike's cardiologist now for over 15 years, I am continually awestruck by his unselfish desire to make the world a better place through his personal actions devoted to this incredibly important cause. Mike's journey from near-death back to life stands as a testament to others faced with the risk of sudden death, and of course to those like Mike who have survived cardiac arrest and face the weight of continued mortality living with a heart disease like HCM. I have no doubt his work will serve as an inspiration to so many of these patients and their families, filling them with the hope and courage necessary to overcome this uninvited adversity, and to have the opportunity to engage life with health and happiness. Mike, thank you.

Martin Maron, MD

Director, HCM Institute, Tufts Medical Center

ONE

The Day I Died

Thursday, August 24, 2006

Sitting in the front row of the bleachers, at age seventeen, without warning, I slumped to the ground. Blackness. Silence. Nothing. I died.

CONOR MEEHAN, seventeen, lowered his gaze from the basketball camp game playing out before him to his best friend suddenly lying at his feet.

"Haha—-very funny, Mike," he muttered, nudging him with his shoe. "Stop messing around."

Mike didn't move. The gym, full of young kids, turned into mayhem. The game stopped.

Realization washed over Conor, and he raced for help. He burst outside the gymnasium doors to find Mike's father, Mike Papale, Sr., in the Wallingford Parks and Recreation Center's lobby. Panic rising, Conor quickly relayed the scene. Mike's dad went white, and he sprinted toward his seventeen-year-old son's lifeless body.

"Mike!" he shouted.

But Mike Papale did not respond. He wasn't breathing. His skin was a ghastly blue. A crowd gathered around the Papales as the chaos continued in the gym. People were running and screaming for help. No one knew what to do—least of all Mike's dad, who watched helplessly as his son lay motionless on the polished floor. Someone called 9-1-1. Another lifted Mike's feet into the air, thinking this might help. Somebody else brought a fan over to try to cool him down. No one realized at the time that Mike was clinically dead—he had suffered sudden cardiac arrest. Cool air and elevated feet would do nothing for him. His only hope to revive was CPR and the shock of an Automated External Defibrillator (AED). But no one knew CPR, and there was no AED onsite. Unbeknownst to those rushing to Mike's aid, with each passing minute his odds of survival dropped precipitously. Statistically, sudden cardiac arrest has a roughly ninety percent survival rate if a shock is administered within one minute. Survival odds plummet another ten percent with each passing minute without defibrillation. Mike was already five minutes post-cardiac arrest.

AT WORK in the building next door, Bob Huebner's pager went off. By chance, the Z-Medica employee and volunteer EMT had set his pager to "scan" that day, to receive emergency alerts. He glanced at the call: *unknown medical, Wallingford Parks and Recreation*. Probably a sprained ankle or bloody nose, he thought. Knowing it takes a while for the ambulance to come across town, he decided to see if he could assist. Strolling through the parking lot, an updated call came: *unconscious teenager on the basketball court*. He started to run. Teens don't lose consciousness unless it's serious.

———

THE PANIC in the gymnasium continued to grow. One of the organizers ordered the gym evacuated. Campers and spectators poured out the doors. The commotion reached John Papale, Mike's thirteen-year-old brother, refereeing a game in the adjacent gym. Bewildered, he made his way through the crowd, led by a sound that would haunt him for years: the chilling screams of his father, pleading, "MIKE!!!"—desperate for a reaction from his son.

———

AT THE PAPALE RESIDENCE, the phone rang. Joan Papale, Mike's mom, picked it up and met a barely recognizable version of her husband's voice. Frantic, quivering, he said, "Come to the rec center right away. It's Mike, and it's bad."

Joan quickly changed, crated the family basset hound, and sped down the driveway.

———

HOPE SLIPPING THROUGH HIS FINGERS, Mike's dad heard a knock on the back door of the gym and ordered another camp employee to open it. The door flew open, smashing Bob Huebner in the head, but it didn't stop him. Bob entered and was surprised by the scene that greeted him. He was quickly brought up to speed, noticing Mike's irregular, almost gasping, breathing. Bob didn't mention it at the time, but what Mike's dad described was agonal breathing--known in the medical world as the last gasps before death. Mike had now been unconscious for almost ten minutes.

Bob immediately took control. He directed a bystander to inform 9-1-1 that there had been a cardiac arrest and to wait outside for the ambulance. He reached for his belt, where, for the past five years, he had worn a CPR holster given to him by a fellow Boy Scout leader, complete with examination gloves and a CPR mask to prevent the transfer of bacteria. Bob began CPR on Mike, hoping it wasn't too late.

Less than a month before, he had completed the American Heart Association Train the Trainer 2005 standards, which educated participants on the new CPR protocol: thirty compressions and two breaths. He knew his job was to keep this up until the medics showed up.

The ambulance arrived eight minutes later and four paramedics hurried to Mike's side to take over. Two began administering oxygen and started an IV delivering careful doses of epinephrine (intended to reverse cardiac arrest by bringing back pulse and blood pressure) and, eventually, amiodarone (to help shock Mike's heart back into rhythm). The other two deftly set up the AED. Bob continued performing CPR. Within seconds, they hit the power button, placed two pads on Mike's chest—on his right just under his collar bone, and beneath his left armpit—and made sure everyone was clear. It was important nobody was touching Mike. Mike Sr. stood by and watched, hopeless and scared. This could not be his seventeen-year old son on the ground seconds from death.

The paramedics delivered the shock. Mike's body

jolted, coming off the ground a few inches. A flat line appeared on the screen.

Seconds later, the flat line crumpled: a heartbeat. Mike's heartbeat. Though he didn't show it, Bob Huebner was overcome with emotion. Mike's heartbeat on that screen instantly became the third most beautiful moment of his life, after the birth of his two sons.

A huge relief, no doubt, but as the EMTs heaved him into the ambulance, Mike was not remotely out of the woods. Between the cardiac arrest and a 150-plus-joule electrical jolt, his heart had endured extreme trauma—not to mention almost twenty minutes of oxygen deprivation. Statistically speaking, his body was likely to revert back to cardiac arrest. Surviving the ride to the hospital would be a significant hurdle.

IF I DON'T HEAR an ambulance, everything is fine, Joan thought as she neared the rec center. Seconds later, a siren wail pierced her soul as an ambulance rocketed past her. Joan saw her husband sitting in the front seat and instantly recognized this as a bad sign. She turned around to chase the ambulance, running red lights, praying to arrive at the hospital and see her son sitting, breathing, talking.

BACK AT THE BASKETBALL CAMP, while John and Conor stood in the lobby struggling to process the morning's events, a police officer walked past and stopped to address the two women working at the front desk.

"I'm here to report a seventeen-year-old male

pronounced DOA (dead on arrival) at Midstate Medical Center after collapsing here this morning."

Numb, speechless, John and Conor felt these words wash over them. They would never speak to Mike again. Mike Papale had died.

TWO

Intensive Care

J oan Papale pulled up to MidState Medical Center in Meriden and reeled internally as she watched Mike being removed from the ambulance, unrecognizable, entwined in ventilator tubes and monitor wires. Joan was in the Twilight Zone.

Inside the hospital, the Papales soon learned that MidState Medical Center would not be Mike's final destination. Upon arrival Mike suffered a second cardiac arrest and was immediately revived by the hospital staff. MMC did not have the proper staff and equipment to keep Mike alive, and he would have to be rushed to Connecticut Children's Medical Center in Hartford, about thirty minutes north.

The initial plan was to transfer Mike via helicopter, but the ER team quickly changed orders to transport him by ambulance. Though the Papales took this as a good sign, the truth was that the helicopter was too small to fit the necessary equipment and personnel to keep Mike alive—which would be tenuous even in an ambulance. Mike was in extremely critical condition.

SPEEDING along the highway toward Hartford, Mike's dad followed behind the ambulance with his mother-in-law, Fayne Kowalski, and Conor's mother, Cindy Meehan, who had met up with the Papales at MidState.

Meanwhile, a dazed Joan sat in the front seat of the ambulance overhearing snatches of conversation from the back. "We may have to paralyze him," floated the voice of one EMT. Moments later, another paramedic peeked her head into the ambulance cab, smiled sympathetically at Joan, and said, "It will be okay." Joan wasn't sure what to believe.

When Mike, still unresponsive, arrived at Connecticut Children's Medical Center, he was raced to the Pediatric Intensive Care Unit (PICU). The unresponsiveness, doctors told the Papales, was partly due to medication and partly to the severe trauma he had just experienced. The Papales stood in a fog as doctors and nurses continued to work on their son.

JOHN AND CONOR eventually arrived at the hospital to find Mike not dead, as the officer had proclaimed at the rec center, but certainly in very serious condition. As they gazed at the unconscious Mike, breathing through a ventilator, they did not know what to say.

That night, Dr. Felice Heller pulled Mike's parents aside and introduced herself. Though the results weren't definitive, and further testing was necessary, she said it was clear Mike had some form of heart disease.

After a stunned silence, Mike's dad erupted. "He can't

have an issue with his heart! He's young, he's in great shape, and he's physically gifted."

Heart conditions, Dr. Heller gently explained, can lie latent in the body and affect anyone—even athletes in the prime of life.

THREE

Coma

Mike's parents didn't sleep that night. John went home with Conor to stay with the Meehans at their house in Meriden. Everyone remained in extreme distress and shock.

Word was spreading like wildfire about what had happened. Nobody could believe it. Home in his living room, watching TV that night, Brandon Gade, a forward on Mike's school and Amateur Athletic Union (AAU) basketball teams, received a call alerting him to the events of the morning and Mike's critical condition. Upset, anxious, and confused, Brandon called several mutual friends to get more details, but nobody knew anything definitive.

The next day—Friday morning—Brandon, his brother Matt, and a bunch of Mike's other basketball teammates piled into a minivan to visit their friend.

The Papales were overwhelmed to see the throng of Mike's friends arrive in the hospital waiting room. One by one, the teammates hugged Mike's parents. Last in line was Brandon. As they embraced, Mike's dad, having served as

Brandon's basketball coach for the previous six years, was overcome with emotion.

"Brandon, it's not good," he said, tears spilling down his cheeks. "I don't know if he's going to make it."

As only two people were allowed into Mike's room at a time, the teammates and friends took turns. No amount of prior conversation about Mike's condition could have prepared them for the moment they first laid eyes on their young friend, lying motionless and unconscious in a hospital bed amid a tangle of medical machinery emitting a steady cacophony of beeps. Two by two they entered the room, only to emerge moments later struggling to process the scene, unsure what to say or do.

No one knew if Mike would wake from his coma. If he would have brain damage. What, specifically, had caused him to suffer this cardiac arrest?

All anyone could do was wait.

FOUR

Awake

Approximately thirty-six hours after his first cardiac arrest, Mike's eyes fluttered open. His face showed a fat lip and a black eye, both injuries caused by the fall he took when he first suffered his sudden cardiac arrest. It was a little after midnight, Saturday, August 26, 2006, and both his parents remained at his side. Though exhaustion gripped Joan, she had not allowed herself to sleep. Seeing Mike's eyes open, she bolted upright and leaned over her son.

"Mom," he said, as he focused on her face. "Dad," he uttered, his eyes finding his father. "Where's John? Is he okay?"

Indescribable relief flooded Mike's parents as they realized he was alive. Alert. And, clearly, *not* braindead. Their prayers had been answered.

"Where am I?" he asked. "Why am I here?"

Joan calmly, gently explained the events of the last day and a half to her son. The end of her story was met with a moment of silence from Mike. And then . . .

"Where am I?" he asked. "Why am I here?"

Mike's parents exchanged a glance of concern, and the medical team soon arrived to re-evaluate their son.

He was suffering from short-term memory loss and disorientation brought on by the trauma. Any questions he asked, any conversation they had, Mike forgot seconds later.

This behavior lasted for a couple of days. Visitors continued to arrive. Mike would recognize them and talk to them, but after they left, he had no memory of seeing them. People sent cards and gifts to the hospital room. John and Conor brought a big card from all the kids that attended the basketball camp. Mike asked Joan if he could read the card. Then he read it to himself. He read each and every name. Then he handed it back to Joan. Five seconds later he asked to read the card again, as if he had never read it before. Joan, terrified Mike would never regain his memory, just went along with it, pretending he had never read the card, and handing it back.

On Sunday morning, the Papales had an early meeting with Dr. Heller and some other doctors. There was serious concern Mike was going to have permanent brain damage. There was still hope his short-term memory would come back, but the doctors thought it should have returned by now. He continued to act confused and agitated. But, when the doctors asked him questions like, "What's your name?" "Where are you?" "What year is it?" Mike could answer all of these questions, which continued to give the doctors and his family hope.

Brandon and Matt came back to visit again, this time with their parents. Mike jokingly said, "Do you have your minivan? Can you sneak me out of here?" Although he still wasn't himself, it was calming to see Mike trying to be funny. Still, everyone was waiting for the moment when he would snap out of it and start acting like himself.

FIVE

Testing
———————

I'm lying in my hospital bed, dazed and confused. My parents are in the room with me. I tell my parents how sore and stiff my body feels. They tell me this is normal since I have been in my hospital bed for days. I have never felt like this before. My body is constantly moving. I never sit still.

When I stretch my legs long, my feet hang off the end of the bed. I look around and see the cards and gift baskets that people have sent me. I have one IV in my arm and one IV on the top of my hand. They don't hurt, but they are uncomfortable. There are electrodes attached to wires on my chest. I look up and see a monitor. The monitor shows my heart rhythm. It shows my heart rate and my oxygen levels.

I have no memory of any of the preceding five days. Though, miraculously, I did *not* die, between my collapse and today, my memory absolutely did. I don't remember visits from friends & family, the conversations I had with them and with the medical staff—nothing.

I have a remote control next to me. It controls the small

TV in the corner of my room. It also has a button to call in the nurse.

The nurse comes in and informs me I'm scheduled to have a cardiac MRI and a surgery to perform a cardiac catheterization later today. I don't even know what this means, but I pretend like I do, and she leaves.

My parents are controlling their emotions. They don't want to scare me. They are happy to see me conscious and remembering things, but they're afraid of what is coming. They recount what happened, narrating the story of my cardiac arrest. They explain the memory loss. I sit and pretend to listen. It's a great deal of information to comprehend. I don't even try to understand it. In fact, I block out the information they tell me. I ignore it. My only focus is the anxiety I feel and how badly my body aches. I keep thinking I'll be heading home soon, and life will go back to normal.

The nurse appears in the door to tell me it's time for my MRI. She wheels me down to the MRI room on my hospital bed. Cardiac Magnetic Resonance Imaging uses a powerful magnetic field, radio waves, and a computer to produce detailed pictures of the structures within the heart. I have to stand up to move from my bed to the MRI machine. I haven't stood in days. I move too fast. I get dizzy. My face turns white. I start sweating and feel weak. I feel like I'm going to collapse. My parents panic and yell to the nurse. Everyone is scared. I just suffered sudden cardiac arrest days earlier. Is it going to happen again? The nurses get me back into my bed and I gradually feel better. I drink some water. The dizziness goes away. Eventually, I get the strength to move, slowly, from my bed to the MRI machine.

I have never had an MRI before. It feels like I'm lying in a coffin, flat on my back, the ceiling just inches from my nose. They give me a damp cloth to put over my face. It doesn't help. I start to sweat. My heart starts to race. I wear head phones to listen to music, hoping this will serve as a distraction, but it doesn't. My entire body is tense. It feels tight. I wish I could be unconscious again so I don't have to feel this pain. The radiologist keeps telling me to hold my breath for an unrealistic amount of time. I think this is ridiculous, but I try my best. I can't do it. They tell me to lie still, but I continue to slightly move my body. They retake image after image because of my movement and my inability to hold my breath. This is never going to end. I feel claustrophobic. More and more sweat is dripping off my body. I feel like I'm in the middle of an endless workout on the hottest day of the year, not an MRI machine. My legs start sticking to the rubber mat I'm lying on. Finally, after three hours, the radiologist takes her last picture and pulls me out of the machine. I take a deep breath of fresh air and feel a huge sense of relief.

The MRI takes much longer than expected, so I'm immediately brought to the operating room for the cardiac catheterization. The doctors explain they are going to use a long, thin, flexible tube called a catheter. They will place the catheter into a blood vessel in my groin and thread it to my heart to remove a small piece of my heart to biopsy. Then, they will examine this specimen under both a regular and an electron microscope. They will put another catheter in a blood vessel in my neck to take two biopsies from the right ventricle of my heart.

I feel like I'm sitting in Spanish class. I don't understand a word they're saying. I nod as if I understand. I don't have a choice.

I wake up after an hour from the surgery, and my stomach is in agonizing pain. I'm having a poor reaction to the anesthesia. I haven't eaten anything all day. I wasn't allowed to eat before the surgery, which helps reduce the risk of vomiting while on the operating table. When I finally do eat, I throw everything up. The hospital food is bad, but not that bad. It's a torturing feeling. Nothing is going in my favor. Nothing feels right.

The final test that day is an echocardiogram, which uses sound waves to create pictures of the heart's chambers, valves, walls, and the blood vessels attached to the heart. This is similar to the test a pregnant woman would get to check on the progress and development of her fetus. Thankfully, this is done right in my hospital room. I don't have to go anywhere. I don't need anesthesia. I'm not getting crammed into a small space. I lie there for thirty minutes as the sonographer jabs the probe, known as a transducer, into my rib cage. I pretend like it doesn't hurt, but every time she pushes the probe into one of my ribs, I wince.

The doctors use the remainder of the day to evaluate the tests and determine a diagnosis. My family and friends stay with me to help the time pass. Later that evening, Dr. Heller reappears in my door. She's ready to deliver the results of the tests.

SIX

Diagnosis

D r. Heller has a warm smile and short, dark hair. She's a pediatric cardiologist and spends a lot of time educating families about how heart disease affects young people. She has delivered test results many times over the course of her medical career, but it never gets easier.

She tells me the left lower chamber of my heart is very thick, and it's conclusive I have a heart disease called Hypertrophic Cardiomyopathy, also known as HCM. My reaction doesn't surprise Dr. Heller. She has seen it before from other young patients. "I can't have heart disease," I tell her. "I'm seventeen-years old. I'm healthy. I'm active. I'm in great shape. I don't smoke. I eat well. Heart disease only affects old people who aren't healthy."

My perception of heart disease is very wrong, she says. HCM is an excessive thickening of the heart muscle, and it's a genetic condition. That means it can affect anyone in my family, including, worst of all, my younger brother.

HCM has a variety of symptoms, including dizziness, shortness of breath, syncope (fainting), chest pain, heart palpitations, and a heart murmur. I have never experienced any of these symptoms. I have, however, experienced the worst possible symptom: sudden cardiac arrest.

HCM is a fairly common disease that affects about one in 500 people across the United States and is the leading cause of death among student-athletes. Each patient suffers differently from the disease, based on the amount of thickening in the heart muscle. Some HCM patients suffer from Hypertrophic Obstructed Cardiomyopathy, or HOCM. Most HOCM patients have a form of the disease in which the wall between the two bottom chambers of the heart becomes enlarged and restricts blood flow out of the heart. Fortunately for me, the doctors did not detect any obstruction. However, in patients that don't have obstruction, the left ventricle of the heart still becomes stiff, which reduces the amount of blood the ventricle can hold and the amount pumped out to the body with each heartbeat. Sometimes, patients with HOCM will experience heart failure and need a heart transplant.

Dr. Heller tells us there is no cure for this condition, meaning I'll be living with this disease for the rest of my life. This leads to the worst news of all: she tells me I'm no longer able to play competitive basketball. I'm seventeen years old, and my basketball career is over. No one is supposed to retire this young. My life-long goal, to play college basketball, has been taken from me. One week ago, I was running to the mailbox each afternoon to grab the envelopes sent to me from college recruiters. Now, I'm sitting in a hospital bed being told I'll never play again. This can't be happening.

While I feel extremely blessed and lucky to be alive, I also feel anger, sadness, and frustration. Why did my basketball career get taken from me? What did I do to deserve this? All the hard work I put in now seems like a waste of time. This isn't fair.

I have a lot of questions for Dr. Heller. Why can't I play basketball? What can I do? Am I going to die younger than I should? How will I stay safe? Can I go back to school? These are just a few. She patiently answers each and every one. She's supportive. She's doing her best to ease my fears. She tries her best to help me believe I can and will live a normal and long life as a Hypertrophic Cardiomyopathy patient.

The doctors work with my family and me to construct a game plan to help me manage my life as an HCM patient. They prescribe a beta-blocker to control heart rhythm, treat chest pain, and reduce high blood pressure.

I meet an electrophysiologist named Dr. Iyer a tall man with dark hair and a charming personality. He's soft spoken but very direct with his words. As he introduces himself, I think, what in the world is an electrophysiologist? An electrophysiologist, he explains, focuses on the heart's timing, or electrical system, to diagnose and treat irregular heartbeats and arrhythmias. He tells me I'll have a defibrillator surgically implanted inside my chest. This sounds complicated. A piece of metal in my chest? The internal cardioverter defibrillator, called an ICD, will sit in a pocket beneath my skin on the left side of my chest, under my collar bone. It has two wires, also known as leads, that will go directly into my heart. The ICD will read my heart rhythm, and, if I experience a dangerous rhythm, it will shock my heart and save my life. I think about what a shock would feel like but don't ask. I don't want to know the answer. The thought alone is painful.

An implanted cardioverter defibrillator runs on a battery. Through check-ups at the doctor's office and a system that will allow me to check my device through the phone, the battery will be carefully monitored. Like any battery, eventually it will run low, and I'll have to get it replaced—but, unlike most batteries, this one requires thoracic surgery to be replaced. The more the device is used, the more energy it will use. Dr. Iyer is hopeful the battery will last seven to eight years before a new one is needed. The only thought that comes to mind as he explains this is that my life will depend on the functionality of a battery.

Dr. Iyer knows I'm afraid. I don't say it aloud, but he knows. He can tell. My face and body language say it all. He knows my parents are just as frightened. He's supportive. He helps me put faith in the ICD. He will perform the surgery, and many of his patients have had great lives following their ICD implantation. He answers all of our questions and tries to help us to look past our concerns and fears.

SEVEN

Surgery: Implantable Cardioverter Defibrillator

I can't sleep. The surgery is in two days, and I'm scared. I lie awake all night thinking. I leave the TV on to distract my mind. I watch re-runs of one of my favorite shows, *The Fresh Prince of Bel-Air*, starring Will Smith. It doesn't help. I lie on my left side and then roll over to my right. Maybe I'll fall sleep if I lie flat on my back. Nothing works. I think about every possible worst-case scenario. I stare at the ceiling, wondering if I'll ever be able to go home. Even when I do, my life will never be the same. I'll always be different than my friends. This is a bad nightmare that I'll never wake up from.

But I don't show my fears. I don't want anyone—my family, my friends, the nurses, or the doctors—to think I'm the least bit afraid. I want them to see how strong I am. But in the back of my mind I'm thinking: How will this piece of metal feel inside of me? Will it affect the motion of my left arm, especially because I'm left-handed? Will I be able to feel the wires going into my heart? What if the device shocks me by mistake? Will it hurt? Will I ever be able to exercise again? I have no idea what to expect. My fear heightens with each minute that passes.

Earlier today, trying to ease my mind, Dr. Iyer assured me that this is a routine surgery, but how routine is any surgery? He explained that with any surgery there are risks, especially when dealing with your heart. Of course, there are!

The plan is to cut a small pocket on the top left side of my chest, under my collar bone, then insert the wires, and attach them to my heart muscle. Then Dr. Iyer will attach those wires to the battery. I wonder, how is this even possible? Dr. Iyer then explained the final step: testing the device. Once the device is properly placed and the incision on my chest is closed, they have to test the ICD to make sure it works properly and effectively. He wants to be assured it's ready to save my life. The medical team will put my body into cardiac arrest, the same rhythm that nearly killed me days earlier.

I wonder, "How does this even make sense?" Why would you want to do that? I got lucky once already. That's enough for a lifetime. They have back up plans in case the device doesn't work, he explained. This is the last step before I can go home, but I can't help but think I'm never going to make it out of this hospital.

As I lie awake, I realize I have to change my mindset. I think about going home. I think about everything going well. I think about my life going forward. But every time I have a positive thought, I think about going into surgery and never waking up.

I stare at the clock and watch each second tick by. It feels like a year has passed, but eventually I see the sun start to rise through my hospital window. I think this could be the last time I see the sun rise. As the minutes pass and the surgery time inches closer, I force myself to think positively. I force myself to believe that my mind can control my body. I accept my situation. My mom tells me I'll never be given a challenge in life that I can't handle. I try to trust what she says. It makes sense, but I'm not sure I can handle this.

Nurses come to my hospital room and wheel me through the hallways to the operating room. My parents walk beside me. I stare at the walls anxiously. I feel cold. For some reason the hallways are way colder than my room. I wonder why that is. I say goodbye to my family as they wheel me into the operating room, which feels like Antarctica. I hate being cold. I tell the medical team how I got sick last time I was under anesthesia and they give me medication to help my stomach. I'm on the operating table, flat on my back. Doctors and nurses stand over me in blue scrubs and masks covering their faces. They are unrecognizable. Who is who? How can I trust these people if I have no clue who they are? What if the doctor had a poor night sleeping, like I did? What if he isn't performing his best today?

I can't think like this. Remember, my mind controls my body. I can handle this situation, just like my mom told me. Slowly, medication is injected into my IV and, from there, into my veins. A coldness runs through my body. The nurses tell me to breathe. I continue to think: I might not wake up. I hope this goes well. Everything is going to be fine.

The nurse tells me to count to ten. 1 . . . 2 . . . 3 . . . and I'm out.

My parents and John are in the waiting area. They are told the surgery will last two hours, so they keep a close eye on the time. The tension is thick. No one says a word. One hour passes. Another hour. No word from the doctor. A third hour passes. My mom is certain something isn't right.

It's now been four hours, double the time the surgery was supposed to last.

Dr. Iyer walks in to the waiting room. His shoulders are slumped. He's moving slowly. He doesn't look happy. My parents' stomachs drop. What could have possibly happened now? With a devastated look on his face, he tells my parents there were complications. The beginning of the surgery went as planned. They implanted the ICD successfully.

Unfortunately, when they attempted to test it, the device did not work properly. Dr. Iyer is not comfortable sending me home like this. He explains to my parents how the ICD can shock at a maximum power of thirty-six joules, but when they test the device, there has to be a ten-joule safety margin. They want the device to work properly on twenty-six joules so they are comfortable it will keep me safe in any situation. He explains how they do the testing knowing the threshold and how there always needs to be a safety margin between the threshold and the maximum available shock strength. He tested the device at twenty joules. It didn't work. He tested the device at twenty-six joules. It didn't work. He tested it again at thirty joules. It worked, but Dr. Iyer is not comfortable with only a six-joule margin of error. I'm stable, and the ICD remains in my chest, but this isn't the end.

I wake up and am immediately told the bad news by Dr. Iyer. How could this happen? At least I didn't die in surgery, I tell myself. But the nightmare continues. I'm beyond frustrated. I want to go home. The complications are delaying my departure from the hospital. This means more long, sleepless nights. How are they going to fix this? How will they protect me from cardiac arrest? Is anything good ever going to happen?

After consulting with multiple doctors throughout the

country, my doctors decide to change my heart medication and "weaken" my heart. "Wait, what?" I ask. My heart is weak as it is. It did just suddenly stop working a little over a week ago, didn't it? Why would they ever want to do such a thing right now? My parents and I are in shock that this is the plan they come up with, but they are the experts, so we agree. They also plan to add a third wire from the device to my heart. This will ensure enough power is generated to shock my heart back, if needed. Just what I want, another surgery.

The next few days are a waiting game. The doctors want to see how my body reacts to the new medicine. Dr. Iyer orders x-rays on my chest to make sure the defibrillator is in the correct location. It is. He wants to be sure my body is ready to endure another surgery without the possibility of infection. My body might be ready, but my mind isn't. The anxiety is back. Although I'm taking medication to lower my heart rate, it skyrockets, pushing 100 beats per minute—and this is while I'm just lying down in bed. The fear is uncontrollable. There is no way positive thinking can fix this.

The night before surgery creeps like an enemy I'm way too familiar with. Another night staring at the ceiling. Another night playing bad scenarios over and over in my head. Another night that feels like years.

I know the routine all too well. The sun comes up. Morning is here. I'm hungry, but I can't eat until after surgery. The nurses wheel me to the operating room. I stare at the walls. My family walks next to me. No one says a word. We all have that same pit in our stomach. This time, it's bigger.

The plan is to test the device once more before surgically implanting a third lead. Dr. Iyer wants to see if the change in medication will solve the issue on its own. There is a chance, the length of the last surgery caused my blood pressure to lower and could be the reason the ICD was not shocking properly. He plans to test the device right away, before there is any drop in blood pressure.

I lie on the operating table, staring up at strangers. It's déjà vu. They're talking to me, trying to ease my mind. Trying to make me feel good. Good try. The thoughts come back.

1 . . . 2 . . . 3 . . . and I'm out.

Dr. Iyer has informed my parents that the procedure will take about two hours again, but warns them there is no guarantee. Again, they sit in the waiting room. Two hours feels like an eternity. No one talks. My parents read. My brother plays his Gameboy. Anything to make time go faster. Anything to get good news.

Twenty minutes pass and Dr. Iyer walks in to greet my parents. This time he has a bounce to his step. He's smiling. My family, surprised to see him so soon, are calmed by his actions. He gives two big thumbs up. They tested the device twice, he tells them. It worked perfectly every time. The doctors were right. Lowering the medication allowed the device to read the rhythms of my heart more effectively. They didn't need to place the third lead. Finally, some good news.

I come out of the surgery, still groggy, with one thing on my mind: going home. The anesthesia is forcing me in and out of sleep, but I feel relief when Dr. Iyer tells me about the successful outcome. The hospital feels like hell on earth. I'm sick of being trapped in a 120 square-foot room on a bed that I don't even fit on. I want to sleep. I want to eat normal food. I want to feel some sort of peace.

After one more day of monitoring me and one more set of x-rays to ensure the device is still placed properly, Dr. Heller walks in and gives me the good news. I can go home. I feel the weight of the world come off my shoulders. I smile. It feels like the first time I've smiled in weeks.

Nurses carefully detach wires from my body. They peel off electrodes from my chest. The beeping sound that I'll forever be able to hear in my head suddenly stops. Dr. Iyer checks the wound from my surgery. There are no signs of infection. They remove the IV from my arm. The irritating IV, one of many that has been placed, removed, and then placed again—gone.

Dr. Iyer, Dr. Heller, my family, and I meet to discuss my treatment plan, which includes 40 milligrams of Nadolol, my beta-blocker, two times per day. I'm ordered to take my medicine when I wake up and when I go to bed. "How long?" I ask. The answer: for the rest of my life. They tell me I have to come back to get checked every three months for the next year. They will reevaluate the frequency of my visits at the end of the year, but for now they want to monitor me closely.

It's hard to focus. It's difficult to remember what they're saying. Thankfully, my mom is diligently taking notes, as she always does. I stare at the doctors, hoping they'll stop talking so we can leave. Finally, they do.

My parents pack up the cards and gift baskets people have sent me. We're lucky to have such a supportive community around us. The nurse shows up with a wheelchair. No way. "There is no chance you are getting me to sit in that thing. I'm walking out of here." Nope – hospital policy. Reluctantly, I sit in the wheel chair, and the nurses slowly walk me down. Through the same hallways I stared at while being wheeled down for surgery. This time, the feeling is different. I don't feel cold. I don't feel anxious. I don't have negative thoughts racing through my mind. I feel good. I feel at peace. I'm happy. I'm ready to move on with my life. We take the elevator down to the first floor of the building.

My dad pulls up the car, and it's waiting when we get downstairs. Seeing our Honda Pilot gives me comfort. The nurses wheel me outside. I take a big breath of fresh air. The air feels good. It's the first time I have been outside in fourteen days. It's a beautiful summer day. The sun is beaming down. The air is warm. I get out of the wheelchair slowly. My body is stiff from lying in a bed for two weeks. I sit in the back seat and we pull away. I turn and look back at the hospital. It gets farther and farther away. I'm more satisfied the farther we get away. Eventually, I can't see it. The place that felt like jail for two weeks is out of sight. Relief courses through my body.

My dad drives forty minutes down Interstate 91 from Hartford to Wallingford. We turn into the driveway and into the garage. I slowly get out of the car. I walk from the garage to the basement, and all of the sudden the anxious feelings are back. I don't feel relieved. I don't feel comfort. I don't feel peace. I'm not happy anymore. I feel anxiety, sadness, confusion, and the worst feeling of all is back: FEAR.

EIGHT

Home

I'm SCARED. But I still refuse to let my parents see how scared I am. They're going through enough with everything that's happened. I can't let my little brother know about my fears either. Two weeks ago, John was told by a police officer I was dead. I have to remain strong for him.

Still, I can't get negative thoughts out of my head. What if I go into cardiac arrest again? What if I go into cardiac arrest and my implanted defibrillator doesn't work? Who is going to monitor my heart every day?

The nurses watching me twenty-four hours a day for the last fourteen days are gone. Those nurses helped me feel safe. As soon as something beeped, someone appeared by my side and fixed it. If I had a question or felt uneasy, I called the nurse and asked. Now I'm home. There are no nurses and no doctors in sight. Neither of my parents are medical professionals.

We eat dinner as a family. Friends have sent food to the house so my parents don't have to cook. I'm happy to be sitting at a kitchen table and not eating hospital food in bed. Everyone is physically and emotionally drained after these two torturous weeks. We don't talk much. The left side of my body feels stiff. I feel the metal. I hope this won't last forever. I hope the feeling goes away and I forget the ICD is there. Bandages cover the wounds where the defibrillator is implanted. Dr. Iyer doesn't want me lifting my left arm over my head for the next few weeks so the ICD can settle into place. I wear a sling on my left arm to remind myself not to lift it. I can only use my right arm. The simple task of cutting my food and eating presents a challenge.

After dinner everyone leaves the table. We're all ready for bed. We go to our rooms. The only thing that has changed, it seems, is the setting. I'm no longer in my 120-square-foot hospital room; I'm in my bedroom. I see the posters hanging on my walls of Michael Jordan and other great NBA players. I look at my trophy case filled with basketball awards I've won. I think about how there will never be another one added. I turn on my TV. I have to lie on my back—lying on my side is off limits because of the sling. Late night re-runs of *The Fresh Prince of Bel Air* play in the background while I stare at the ceiling.

I remember being told sudden cardiac arrest can happen at any time, even during sleep. I can't get that thought out of my head. Finally, I'm home. I'm able to sleep in my own bed. I've been waiting for this moment every night I laid in my hospital bed staring at the ceiling. Now, I'm afraid to sleep in my own bed. I'm afraid that, if I go to sleep, I'll never wake up. I think about dying in my sleep. I ponder how I won't even know the difference if it happens. Then I think, if I don't go to sleep, I can't die in my sleep. I'm safe if I don't actually fall asleep.

I think about the limitations on my life right now. The biggest is not being able to play basketball, but right now I also can't run, can't drink or eat anything with caffeine, and I can't lift weights. I'm an active person. I like playing all types of sports with my friends. Will I ever be able to do that again? I force myself to stay awake. I can't go to sleep. I don't care how tired I am. I can't die in my sleep. Not tonight. My parents cannot come in my room tomorrow morning to find me dead in my bed. I won't let that happen. They have been through enough to last a lifetime. I stay awake. Eventually the sun starts to peer in through the curtains. Finally, a new day.

My senior year of high school has started, but my doctors have given me strict instructions to stay home until I see them in a week for my first follow-up appointment. All week I talk to my friends about their days and I get jealous. I wish I could go to school. I wish I could hang out in the hallways between class. I miss interacting with teachers. My life doesn't feel real right now.

My parents do their best to get me out of the house. They take me out to lunch and to visit my friends. I go on walks around the neighborhood to get fresh air. I'll do anything to help pass the time. I spend the majority of my days on the couch watching TV, something I don't love to do. My once crazy and hectic lifestyle has completely slowed down. I need to get my life back.

NINE

Before I Collapsed

I was born in Wallingford, Connecticut, a town of approximately 45,000 people right in the middle of the state, between New Haven and Hartford. My mom was very passionate about academics. Both her parents were teachers. She thought she was destined for law school, but her path changed and she became a teacher as well. My dad was passionate about athletics. He was a star athlete growing up and excelled in football, basketball, and baseball. He played basketball and baseball at Assumption College, where he's a member of their athletics Hall of Fame. He was the Head Varsity Basketball Coach at Sheehan High School when I was born.

My parents instilled core values in John and me from a young age. They taught us the importance of hard work and being a good person. They never forced us to do anything. They let us follow our own passions. My dad had a deep love for basketball, but he never forced it on John or me. It was expected that we worked hard in everything that we did, especially in school. My parents did not accept bad grades, and if we did receive a bad grade, we needed to offer an explanation and reach out to our teacher to figure it out.

I started playing basketball when I was six years old. At first, I was a bit unsure about the game. I didn't love it. I wasn't aggressive. I didn't want to touch the ball. I ran up and down the court, hoping no one passed it to me. My dad didn't care. He let me know I could do whatever I wanted to do.

My attitude toward basketball quickly changed when my parents put a small basketball court in our backyard so I could practice and play any time I wanted to. I grew rapidly, becoming one of the tallest kids in my grade, and my basketball skills quickly followed.

My parents didn't put pressure on me, but I put pressure on myself. I didn't understand how to lose. I got angry and showed my emotions on the court. If the referee made a bad call, I would slam the ball on the ground. If someone on my team made a mistake, I lashed out at them. My parents quickly put an end to this behavior. They taught me how to control these negative emotions. They forced me to write letters, apologizing to referees and wouldn't let me play in the next game if I yelled at a teammate. They knew how much it hurt me to be forced not to play. It instantly reversed my behavior.

Basketball became an obsession. I spent hours in our backyard or in gyms honing my skills. Losing only fueled my fire. I couldn't accept other kids beating me. If I lost, I worked harder. Instead of pouting or yelling, I spent my time improving my skills, so the next time I faced this opposition I came out with a victory. My parents let me practice as much as I wanted, as long as it did not impact my grades in any way.

My father founded Hoop House Basketball Camp before my brother and I were born. The camp served boys and girls ages six to sixteen and was one of the highlights of the summer for John, Conor, and me. Conor and I met at the camp when we were seven years old, playing in a game against each other. Conor had the same competitive spirit that I had. We both thought we were the best, and neither one of us wanted to lose. When Conor hit a game winning shot to beat my team, I was devastated. How could I lose to this kid I'd just met? In that moment, I hated him. I hated losing, and he'd taken a win away from me. We were just seven-years old, but it felt like I'd lost to my lifelong rival. Shortly after the game, the counselors moved me up to the older division. Who cares about losing now? I got to move up and play with the older kids, and Conor had to play with the little kids. We've been best friends ever since.

Conor and I played on the same travel team during the winter and AAU team during the spring and summer. Every day that we weren't in school, we hung out together. He came to my house or I went to his. Most of the time we just played basketball. As we grew, we both had a common goal: to play in college. My dad, who coached us both, was clear that we had to work very hard to make this happen. We understood the hard work and dedication needed to reach our goal.

Conor and I worked out every day in the summer. Our parents dropped us off at local gyms in the morning with ten dollars for lunch. We spent hours working out. We did ball handling drills, shooting drills, played one on one, and worked on our conditioning. We were both competitive, especially with each other. Everything we did had to have a winner and a loser. The winner boasted and the loser was angry. We were best friends, but there was no one we hated losing to more than each other. After hours of working out, we always walked to our favorite place for lunch, Vinny's Deli, to have a sandwich and a chocolate chip cookie. After lunch, we went back to the gym to work out more. We went home to rest, eat dinner, and then went to our AAU practice at night. It was basketball all day and all night for both of us. Nothing was better.

When we reached high school age, we went to different schools. He attended Choate Rosemary Hall, a college preparatory school in Wallingford, and I attended Xavier High School, an all-boys Catholic school in Middletown.

At Xavier, I earned some minutes as a freshman on the varsity team. As a sophomore, we had a really good team, and I earned a starting role. At the end of the year, I started to find myself unhappy. I didn't love the school anymore. I wasn't excited by the atmosphere. I didn't have a great relationship with the other players on the team. Our team was successful, but I didn't have the same joy playing there that I had playing basketball in the past. Basketball was my true love in life and when I started feeling unhappy playing there, I knew it was time for a change. I decided to transfer back to Sheehan High School, one of the public schools in Wallingford.

The guys I'd played basketball with in middle school were thrilled. The coach, who had taken over after my dad left, was excited to have me back playing for his team.

Due to the transfer rules, I was able to practice with the team, but I was not allowed to play until the eighth game of the year. It was the first time I had to sit on the sidelines.

Finally, the day came, and we were playing against our cross-town rival, Lyman Hall High School. I sat in my room before I left for the game, reading a book about

Michael Jordan. It motivated me. Michael Jordan was my hero.

The bleachers were packed with fans from town. Both student-sections were filled. I was nervous and excited at the same time. As we warmed up, the Lyman Hall student section chanted "Over-rated" at me. It just added fuel to the fire. I was nervous before the game but I didn't allow it to show. I wanted my teammates to have confidence in me. It was an exciting game that went back and forth the entire time. We gained a lead in the fourth quarter and held onto it for a close victory. I scored twelve points in my first game back and had one of the highlights of my season throwing a "no look" pass to one of my teammates who finished the play by scoring a lay-up under the basket. Our fans reacted to the exciting play with a loud roar. We had a great season and I was our team's leading scorer. We went into the state playoffs as an underdog and won three games against teams ranked higher than us. We eventually lost to Torrington High School in the state semi-finals. Torrington won the state championship that year.

After the high school season ended, Conor and I were back in the gym. We were both happy with our high school seasons, but we weren't satisfied. The goal was to play basketball in college, but neither of us had gotten recruited yet. We had a big summer ahead. We had to be prepared, because our AAU team was scheduled to attend various showcase tournaments in front of college coaches.

We spent the summer traveling to tournaments all throughout the Northeast and down to Florida. At each game, college coaches surrounded the court, watching us closely, trying to find a player who was good enough to take their team to the next level.

I was nervous. I'd spent hours in the gym for this moment, but what if I wasn't good enough? What if none of these coaches thought I was good enough to play for them? If none of these coaches liked me, my dream wouldn't come true. On top of winning and losing, this added pressure to every game.

I played well that summer. I was known as a combo-guard, a guard that can be both a point guard and a shooting guard. I was a lethal three-point shooter. It was the best part of my game.

The summer passed very quickly. We played our last tournament at AAU Nationals in Orlando, at Disney's Wide World of Sports Complex. It was our last chance to get seen by college coaches. The pressure mounted in each game to not only win, but to play well.

Some coaches took notice. When the tournaments ended, my cell phone started to ring. College coaches were telling me why I should attend their school. Each day I ran to the mailbox to find stacks of letters from colleges all over the Northeast. My parents' emails were flooded with college coaches reaching out to them. Some of the best Division Two and Division Three schools throughout the country wanted me.

I took a strong liking to Trinity College, which competes in the New England Small College Athletic Conference (NESCAC). Coincidentally, Conor was being heavily recruited by Amherst College, which competes in the same conference. Our dream was coming true.

Hoop House Basketball Camp was at the end of summer that year, the second-to-last week before my senior year started. Conor, John, and I were all counselors at camp. John was heading into eighth grade, where he was the star of his middle school basketball team. Conor and I continued to train. We were getting recruited, but that didn't mean it was time to stop, and John was right behind us every step of the way.

On Wednesday evening, John and I decided we'd wake up early the next morning and work out before camp started. This way, once the day was over, we could relax and enjoy the summer night. We called one of our friends, Jeremy, who liked to put us through various drills. He agreed to pick us up the next morning at 6:30 a.m.

The next morning, Thursday, August 24, John and I woke up and ate our breakfast. Nothing seemed out of the ordinary. We waited eagerly in the living room until Jeremy's blue SUV pulled up in front of our red colonial house. We walked outside, locked the front door, and were off to Choate Rosemary Hall to start our workout.

Jeremy always requested we bring a notebook to keep track of the shots we took and how many of them we made. This allowed us to chart our progress over time. The workout started. We took shots with one hand from close and slowly moved back. Quickly we transitioned to ball handling drills. We spent time sprinting to half-court before sprinting in and shooting three-pointers. John and I were drenched with sweat. It was pouring off of us, but we felt fine. We had done these drills hundreds of time before. Nothing was different about today. The workout lasted ninety minutes.

Afterwards, we hopped back into Jeremy's SUV and drove to the Wallingford Parks and Recreation Center to work the camp. Thursday was always contest day, a fun day where the kids competed against their team in a variety of different drills. There was one winner for each team. The winners would then compete against the rest of the camp the next day.

We pulled up Fairfield Boulevard, and Jeremy dropped us off at the front door of the Recreation Center. I went to the athletic trainer's room to change my shirt. I said, "What's up?" to my dad. I ordered my lunch for later. It was 8:15 a.m. That's the last thing I remember from that day.

I put the kids through the contests, I coached a game, I took the kids outside to do drills—but I don't remember any of it.

TEN

Meeting My Hero

My parents announce we have an appointment at the firehouse in town. They tell me we're going to meet our heroes, the people who saved my life. I feel grateful toward these people, but I'm not sure I'm ready to meet them right now. It sounds awkward. It sounds emotional. I don't like to display my emotions. But I don't have a choice. The decision is made. We're going.

My parents, John, and I drive ten minutes through town and arrive at the firehouse. There are people waiting outside. One guy is dressed in street clothes. The other four, three men and a woman, are in uniform. They are standing there, eagerly, with big smiles on their face. Often, EMS workers don't even know if their patients survive and make it out of the hospital, let alone meet them. This isn't just a special day for us; it's a special day for them.

I'm nervous. I wonder, what do you even say to someone who saved your life? Is saying thank you enough? I sure hope so because I don't know what else to say.

Bob Huebner is the man in street clothes. As I look at

him, I think about the day of my cardiac arrest. What if one thing had gone differently? What if Bob had been sick that morning? What if he hadn't had his pager on? What if he'd been traveling for work and not in the office? Simple answer: I would have died.

My dad pulls the car into a parking spot. The doors unlock. My anxiety rises. I have no clue how this is going to go. I walk up to Bob and do what my parents taught me to do any time I meet a stranger. I put my hand out to shake his hand. He puts his hand out, firmly grips my hand, and pulls me in for a hug.

Bob is about six feet tall with short hair. He has a big smile and a round face. He wears his cell phone on his belt clip. I notice something else on his belt. I don't know it at the time, but it's a CPR holster, similar to the one he used to save my life. In a tan shirt and dark shorts with white New Balance sneakers, he's a regular guy but, to us, he looks like Superman. He saved our world.

Bob says, "Last time we were together, my mouth was on your mouth."

Everyone laughs. Thankfully, with that one statement, Bob eases the tension for all of us. My parents hug him. They don't want to let go. My parents are crying. Bob is crying.

I try not to cry. It's uncomfortable watching my parents cry. I don't like seeing them like this. I understand these are tears of joy, fear, relief, and respect. My parents know that, without Bob's knowledge of CPR, their son would not be standing here. If not for this man, the tears of happiness would have been tears of unbearable sadness. I can't begin to imagine what that day was like for them. I can't imagine what that day was like for John. They deserve to cry as much as they need to.

Once we meet everyone, and the emotions have

subsided, they give us a tour of their facility and talk to us about the training they go through. I am able to relax now. I enjoy talking to them. They make my family and me smile and laugh. It's amazing. I realize how important this day is for them. These people, basically strangers, care so much for my family and me. They are elated we're there with them. They don't want us to leave. There's a connection between us that is indescribable. It feels like we've known each other for years. They're so happy to see me sitting in front of them. Breathing. Talking. Laughing. The last time they saw me, I was near death.

We spend a few hours sharing stories, exchanging memories, and talking about life. As we shake hands to say goodbye, there is a connection between us. A bond that cannot be broken.

ELEVEN

Genetics

When Dr. Heller told us in the hospital that Hypertrophic Cardiomyopathy is a genetic condition, we were stunned. Who else has it? My father or mother has to have it, right? Will John get it?

I have been home from the hospital for over a week, and it's time for my family to get tested. It's highly likely one of my parents has HCM and just doesn't know it, so they go together to the hospital to get an electrocardiogram and an echocardiogram.

The results are clear immediately. My mom's tests are negative. No signs of excessive thickening in her heart muscle. My dad's, however, are positive. We all wonder, how has he been living with HCM his entire life? He's completely asymptomatic. This doesn't make sense. I went into cardiac arrest at seventeen. My dad, at age forty-five, has no symptoms. He's an athlete. He still plays sports. How is his life going to change now? This doesn't seem fair to him. How could a disease that has never affected him change his life so much?

The doctors tell him he's considered a high-risk

patient. If one family member has gone into sudden cardiac arrest, it makes others in the family showing the disease high-risk. They urge my father to have an ICD placed immediately. They tell him he needs to start taking beta blockers right away. Sudden cardiac arrest can happen at any time, and he needs to be safe. There is no other way to protect him.

But my father decides against this treatment. This disease has never affected him. Why would anything happen now? He's scared. What if something happens in surgery? What if the medicine has side effects?

My mom and I do everything we can to change his mind. We find different doctors and they try to convince him to move forward with this. Nothing works. He won't budge. Finally, we give in. Though frustrated and confused, I force myself not to be mad at him. It's his life, and he has to make his own decision.

John is next in line to get tested. He's thirteen years old. There is no way he can have this disease, is there? My parents set up an appointment with Dr. Heller. I can't go. I'm too fearful of what the results could be. I won't be able to handle it if John tests positive. I don't want to see his reaction. His heartbreak. My little brother doesn't deserve to have this happen to him. He's too young to have his basketball career end now.

My parents and John go to the hospital. I stay home by myself, feeling sick. I just want the news that his results are negative. I'm doing anything I can do to make time speed up. I watch TV. It doesn't work. I listen to music. It doesn't work. I go for a walk. Time is moving slow. It feels like they've been at the hospital for days, weeks, and I'm suffering as I wait to hear the news.

My cell phone rings. I want to throw up. I pick up the

phone. My mother is on the other line. He doesn't have HCM . . . for now.

Dr. Heller tells my parents that John is not in the clear. Often times, HCM won't show itself until the later teenage years, so there's still a chance that John will develop the disease. We have two options. John can get tested every year and be monitored very closely, or we can try genetic testing. Genetic testing is the process of taking a sample of a person's DNA to look for changes that can cause heart disease. These changes are called pathogenic, or disease causing, mutations.

My parents decide it makes the most sense to give the genetic testing a chance. I'm the first person who needs to get tested. They need to isolate the gene that's causing my HCM.

There are three types of results that can occur after the initial person is tested. A positive result means the laboratory is confident it has identified a gene mutation causing HCM. A negative result means the laboratory was unable to find a mutation capable of causing disease in any of the genes evaluated. The third result is a genetic variant of uncertain significance. This means there are changes in DNA, but the laboratory is unable to determine if these changes are the cause of the HCM. We're hoping for a positive result from my test. If my test has a positive result, the laboratory will be able to test John's DNA for that same gene, ultimately determining if he's at risk to develop HCM.

I go to the doctor and they take some bloodwork. By now I should be immune to being poked and prodded with needles, but watching the doctor pull the needle out of the plastic still gives me that harrowing feeling. I never look when they insert the needle. It makes me uncomfortable. I don't want to see blood coming out of my own body.

Finally, they collect the blood they need to send to the laboratory. It will take six to eight weeks for the results. Another waiting game.

A couple of months later, Dr. Heller calls my house to talk to my mom. The results are in. They can't isolate my gene. They didn't get the positive result. The test results in a genetic variant of uncertain significance. John is stuck in the gray area. He might develop the disease, he might not. We won't know. He will get tested every year.

John is young but this uncertainty puts fear in the back of his mind. He can live his life normally, but he knows there is a chance his life will change with one doctor's appointment. We don't talk about this with each other. Neither one of us are comfortable talking about it. John doesn't show a lot of emotion, but he is anxious.

I think about how I felt the day of his initial testing. It felt like torture. How am I going to handle this every year? What if he develops the disease in between tests? He could go into cardiac arrest without us knowing about the disease. Everything feels like an unknown for John. I hate that feeling. I want to know one way or the other. Unfortunately, I don't have a choice.

TWELVE

Giving Back

I'm sitting in my room watching TV with my door closed. I hear a knock on the door. It's my mom. I tell her to come in and she seems happy and excited. She tells me about a meeting she's set up for us. She hasn't even told me what it is yet, but like any teenager, I know I probably don't want to go. She then tells me the meeting is at the American Heart Association. They have an office in town, and they want to meet me. They want to hear my story. Now I *definitely* don't want to go.

I'm a very shy person. I don't talk to people I don't know well. I especially hate talking in front of groups. I don't want to tell these strangers what happened to me. I make my case as to why I don't think we should go. "I'm fine now. Let's move on with our lives, please. Let's just put this behind us forever."

My mom offers her rebuttal and I quickly learn I'm not going to win this battle. She explains to me how I can make an impact, I can make a difference. My story is powerful. I can help raise awareness about heart disease, about CPR, and about AEDs. I'm lucky to be alive and this is my chance to give back. I can *save lives*.

I can see this is important to my mom, so I agree to go.

The next morning, we drive to the American Heart Association office. Upon entering, we're greeted by two employees, Robert Townes and Lisa Franco, who are very excited to see me. I don't know much about their work, but they explain how the AHA is a nonprofit organization that spends every day trying to save people of all ages from dying of heart disease and stroke. They tell me I'm the reason they come to work every day. They are familiar with my story and are inspired.

They ask me to tell my version of the story. I tell to them everything I remember, and then I reiterate everything I've been told. As I speak, their faces light up. They grow taller in their chairs. My attitude about the meeting suddenly changes. I'm happy to be here. I'm pleased to be sharing my story with these strangers. Something feels really good about this. If my story can have this type of an impact on these two people, maybe I really can make an impact on others. That seems cool. Never in my life have I ever though about making a difference in the world.

Then they ask my mom to tell her version. I've never heard her talk about what happened that day and how it affected her. As she talks, I want to cry, but I hold back the tears. It's not my fault, but I feel terrible for what she went through. She received the phone call no parent ever wants to get: something is terribly wrong with your child. She drove to the hospital not knowing if I would be dead or alive when she arrived. I can feel her emotions, her pain. I can also feel her passion. She doesn't want any mother to have to go through what she did. She doesn't want any parent to get that phone call. After listening to my mom talk, my inspiration to make a difference is soaring. I feel motivated. I want to share our story. I know my mom wants this more than anything, and I want to be there with her every step of the way. I want to save lives.

The American Heart Association asks us if we will serve as volunteers and spokespeople for them. They want to use our story to help fulfill their mission. Our story is the reason they do the work that they do. My mom and I don't even have to think about it. We're all in. We sign some paperwork allowing them to use my story, my name, and my picture.

As my mom and I walk out of the office and into the car, I feel differently than I have for the past few weeks. I thank my mom for setting up the meeting. I tell her I envision myself working for the American Heart Association someday.

When basketball was taken from me, I felt like I lost my purpose. I felt like I had no goals to work for. I wasn't sure why I even existed anymore. I feel this starting to change. I feel like I have a different purpose now.

THIRTEEN

Finding My Way

I have been at home, recovering, for two weeks. I've missed a lot of school and I'm way behind on assignments. I'm starting to get antsy at home. There is only so much I can do to keep myself occupied. My friends are all talking about school and the fun they're having. I feel left out and want to get back to my normal schedule.

My teachers meet with me to discuss an action plan to get caught up with all the work I've missed and to set up a plan in case my ICD shocks me. They're all understanding and happy to see me healthy and doing well.

Brandon picks me up for school on my first day. I feel a little bit nervous. The negative thoughts start to come back. What if I go into sudden cardiac arrest in the hallway between classes? What if no one knows what to do? How will I survive?

I walk into school and people are staring at me like I'm a celebrity. Mr. Ainsworth, my junior year Algebra teacher, sees me immediately, and asks how I am feeling. My friend Steve comes up to me and gives me a big hug. He visited me multiple times in the hospital and is excited to see me in a different setting. Members of the basketball team give me a pat on the back. Everyone is nice. Everyone is happy to see me. Word has spread around town about what happened. People start to ask questions, and I tell them everything. I don't like the attention, but I don't have a choice. Teachers are keeping a close eye on me. Everyone wants to make sure I'm feeling okay. I keep telling everyone that I'm fine.

I slowly catch up with my school work and get back into the flow of things. I get a routine back. It's nice. I enjoy the structure of going to school every day.

Before my near-death, I never worried about my diet. I enjoyed my fair share of fast food and dessert, just like any other high school student. When I was playing basketball, I burned so many calories, between working out and playing games, that I was able to eat anything. My body always looked great, and I was proud of that. But I'm not exercising at all right now—I'm afraid to. I don't want to do anything to increase my chances of another sudden cardiac arrest. I don't want my implanted defibrillator to go off. But I still savor fast food from time to time. I still indulge in dessert. I don't gauge my carbohydrate intake. It's never mattered before. Why should it matter now?

One morning, as I get out of the shower and start to get dressed for school, I look in the mirror. My body looks different. It isn't as cut as it once was. It looks like I gained weight. I step on the scale and it reads 220 pounds. I was 190 pounds before my cardiac arrest. Something has to be wrong. The scale has to be broken, right? I never gain weight. I have to work hard to even put weight on. Not anymore.

Suddenly, I feel self-conscious. I hate the way I look. I'm embarrassed by it. Am I the only one who's just noticing this? I wonder what everyone else is thinking. Just over a month ago, I was ripped—you could count my abs. Now you can't even see them. I put on a baggy shirt, hoping no one will detect my weight gain.

Later that day, the bell rings, and I'm heading to my next class—physical education. My stomach drops. I don't want to change in front of my classmates. I don't want them to see what I saw earlier this morning. I'm certain they'll laugh at me, will think less of me. They'll call me fat behind my back. The long walk through the hallways to the locker room reminds me of the commute from hospital room to operating room. I already can barely participate in gym class—I have too many restrictions. But the thought of changing in front of people? I don't even want to take my shirt off.

Worst of all, we're transitioning to start the swimming section of P.E. There is no way I'm getting in that pool. Not only are the boys going to see me change, but the girls are going to see me shirtless in the pool? No way. I tell my teachers I'm not allowed to be swimming right now because of my heart. It's a complete lie, and I feel terrible about it. How can I use my heart disease as an excuse to get out of something I don't want to do? But I don't care. Anything so I don't have to take my shirt off in front of my peers.

FOURTEEN

Shifting My Path

I had dedicated my life to basketball. I worked so hard. My dream was coming true. I was so close. Now, it's over. My basketball career is over forever.

I think back to my junior year of high school and the run to the state semi-finals. I played four of the best basketball games of my career, averaging twenty-six points per game in the tournament. I was starting to hit my prime. None of that matters anymore. I'm never playing basketball again.

I have a very hard decision to make. Do I want to even be around the game anymore? Will it just make me sad that I can't play? Maybe I should just put basketball in the past and move on with my life. Or, maybe there are other ways to enjoy basketball without playing. I'm not ready to make this decision, but it feels like I have to.

John is starting to evolve as a player. He's the best athlete on the Moran Middle School team and is playing AAU basketball in the spring. He has the potential to be one of the best young players in the state of Connecticut, even better than I was. For this reason, I can't leave basketball behind. It's still a huge part of my life. I want to watch John. I want to help him. I want to see his career unfold. He always tagged along with my friends and me, always played with us. We were always bigger and stronger, but that didn't matter. He was always there, ready to play.

The decision is made for me. Basketball is still going to be a big part of my life. If I can't play, I can watch my brother. I can help him. If I'm not be able to be a basketball player, maybe I can be a basketball *coach*.

Joe Gaetano, my high school coach at Sheehan, has been very supportive of my family and me. He came to visit me multiple times during my stay in the hospital and told me he still wanted me to be involved with the team. He asks me to be a student-assistant. I can attend all the practices and sit on the bench in a shirt and tie during the games. This is my first opportunity to coach.

At first, I hate it. I sit on the bleachers during our first team practice. I watch my peers run up and down the court, working on their skills and executing the plays. I don't say anything. The coaches urge me to stand up, closer to the sideline to get a better view. I should be out there playing, I think. I worked my whole life for this. I can help the team win. I can't help from the sideline. I'm useless here.

Eventually, I start to be more vocal. I don't just stand on the sidelines. I yell and encourage my teammates who are on the floor. I correct them when they make a mistake. I encourage them when they feel unsure. I start to feel like I have a purpose on the sidelines.

Each year, a variety of players from each state are nominated for the McDonald's All-American game. The amount of nominations per state depends on the size of the state. Out of all of the nominations throughout the country, only twenty-four are selected to actually play in the game. These are typically the top twenty-four players in the entire country who are headed to play high level Division One basketball and eventually in the NBA. The nominations are based upon a player's junior year performance. I find out that I'm one of six players nominated in Connecticut. Conor is also nominated. It's an honor to share such a prestigious award with my closest friend.

Conor's basketball career continues to progress. He's getting recruited by schools at the Division One, Division Two, and Division Three levels, but he has his mind set on Division One and doesn't want anything else.

Word continues to spread about what happened to me. There is shock and sadness from many. I receive an incredible amount of support from people throughout the state. I also receive tons of phone calls from different local newspapers, like The *Record Journal* and the *New Haven Register,* looking to write stories about my cardiac arrest. Reporters start coming to our practices at Sheehan to talk to me, even though I'm not even playing. I hate the attention. It's not fair to my teammates. They are on the court, working hard every single day in practice. How am I the one getting publicity?

It's an up and down season for our team. We're winning some games and losing some. Our schedule is challenging. I feel better about my role and am doing my best to help the team. The players rely on me. They respect my opinion. They talk to me. They ask me why I think they missed their last shot or how they can do a better job guarding the person they're defending.

Watching the high school team play is hard, but attending games at the local YMCA on the weekends is even worse. Conor and I spent our lives going to the Meriden and Wallingford YMCA to play pick-up basketball. I still go with him, but now I have to sit on the side as a spectator and watch him play. I know I hate being there, but I can't stop going. The gym is where I belong, and Conor is my best friend. I want to spend time with him. This is what we do together—we go to the gym. I desperately want to get out there on the court, but I know I can't risk my life.

FIFTEEN

Volunteering

I have fun volunteering for the American Heart Association. It gives me purpose. They're using my picture everywhere. I'm a walking advertisement for why CPR and AEDs are important. People must wonder how this young kid has heart disease. I used to think that way too. Not anymore.

The first big event we participate in is the annual New Haven Heart Walk, where the AHA highlights me as a survivor. They invite me to cut the ribbon to start the walk. It's a great atmosphere. A DJ is blasting music. People are dancing and playing yard games in a huge field. The race is about to start, and I see a group of guys walking toward me. I soon realize it's all of the kids from my AAU basketball team. They surprise my family and me to show us support. Having them there makes the day that much better. This is the first time I've seen a lot of them since my release from the hospital.

Later that year, the American Heart Association invites my family and me to Washington, D.C., to lobby Congress about heart disease, sudden cardiac arrest, and the importance of CPR and AEDs. We feel honored. We're making a difference in Connecticut, but imagine the impact we can have in the nation's capital.

We drive six hours south to D.C. to attend the opening ceremonies for the event and hear from a variety of inspiring speakers advocating for heart health. The next day, my mom and I attend a "Go Red for Women" event. This event is used to raise awareness of how heart disease affects women across the country. The AHA started this initiative because they determined heart disease was taking the lives of more than 500,000 women across the United States each year, and people were not paying enough attention to it. The national consensus is that heart disease is an "old man's disease." The goal of this initiative is to empower women to take charge of their heart health. It's inspiring to see the number of people in attendance, all dressed in red, trying to help save lives.

Later that afternoon, we're sent to different buildings to talk to Congress about our story. This is my first time in Washington, D.C., and I'm in awe of the different buildings. They have tall columns, triangular pediments, and symmetrical shapes. The marble statues and glass walls inside each building are breathtaking. I wear a black suit with a bright red tie, making it clear I'm there to advocate for heart health. I don't wear suits often, but for some reason I feel important dressed in this one. There's something special about walking around the streets of Washington, D.C. in a suit and tie.

All day we're surrounded by people, both younger and older, who also have stories of survival or are living with heart disease. Sadly, some of the parents we're with have lost a child to sudden cardiac arrest. The American Heart Association is focusing on four main issues throughout the day. These issues are to increase funding for heart disease and stroke research and prevention at the National Institutes of Health (NIH), to increase funding for heart disease and stroke research and prevention at the Centers for Disease Control and Prevention (CDC), to lobby for The HEART for Women Act which will improve the prevention, diagnosis, and treatment of heart disease, stroke, and other cardiovascular diseases in women, and to lobby for The STOP Stroke Act which will ensure that stroke is widely recognized by the public and treated more effectively by health care providers.

In each meeting, we're greeted by a different member of Congress. We meet with Senators Joseph Lieberman and Chris Dodd, but the highlight of the day is meeting with Rosa DeLauro, the U.S. Representative for Connecticut's Third Congressional District. In her carefully decorated office are pictures that serve as a visual biography of her career. She seems excited to see us. Her bright and vibrant clothes match her dynamic personality. She focuses in on each and every one of us as we share our personal experiences. She seems interested. She asks questions. She wants to help us with our mission.

We're heading into our last meeting of the day. Each building is equipped with heavy security at the door. There are armed officers and metal detectors, and no one can enter without going through a metal detector or getting frisked by one of the security guards.

We wait in a long line, and it's almost my turn. I take my belongings out of my pockets, and all of a sudden, the officers are screaming. Everyone needs to leave the building. The building is being evacuated. There's a potential threat. We quickly exit and walk away from the building. I turn around and see officers armed with automatic weapons—huge machine guns, the ones you see in movies. This is scary. Six years prior were the September 11 terrorist attacks. They are still fresh in our minds. We later learn the evacuation was due to a precautionary measure —there was no real threat—but we didn't stick around long enough to find out.

The family trip in Washington, D.C., flies by. The ride home is quiet. We're all tired. We drive through Pennsylvania into New Jersey and eventually New York. Finally, we cross the Connecticut border. We start to talk about how inspired we're by the trip. Our family really can make a difference.

I have an idea. We should start our own organization someday. But it doesn't seem possible. How would we pull it off? Where do we even start? I never thought it would be possible for me to have a dream that didn't involve basketball. We pull into our garage. My basketball career might be over, but my life is just beginning.

SIXTEEN

Treatment

I visit Dr. Heller and Dr. Iyer every three months and they tell me my treatment is going well. I'm never excited to go back to the hospital, but I do like being around these doctors. I know how crucial their role was in saving my life and keeping me safe. We get along well. I appreciate how much they care about me. They consider how I'm feeling, both physically and mentally.

Dr. Heller always orders an electrocardiogram and an echocardiogram. It's important to monitor the thickening of my heart muscle. If it continues to thicken, I might start to develop day-to-day symptoms as well as other complications, eventually including heart failure. We're pleased to hear at each appointment that the thickening hasn't changed.

Dr. Iyer's appointment is different. I get my ICD interrogated. I sit in chair while a nurse from St. Jude (now Abott), the company that manufactures my ICD, prepares the interrogation. The nurse takes a wand, attached to a computer, and places it over my ICD. All of a sudden, my name pops up on the computer screen, and the programming of my device appears. My heart rhythms also appear, showing my heart rate: fifty-three. This is normal for me because of the effects the beta blocker has on my body. My resting heart rate is lower than the average person's. I see a button that says *shock* and think, whatever you do, don't put your finger near that button! There is a bar filled to about 85% in green—my battery level. I don't feel like a human. I feel like a machine. A machine running on a battery.

The nurse tells me she wants to test the settings of my ICD to make sure it recognizes my heart rate. She says I'm going to feel my heart start to race. She presses a button. I see the number on the screen representing my heart rate skyrocket. Sixty-five. Eighty. Ninety. It keeps going. Then I feel it. My heart is racing like I'm sprinting up and down the basketball court, but I'm not—I'm sitting in a chair in an exam room. For a moment my heart feels like it's going to explode out of my chest. Then the nurse presses another button and my heart rate starts to lower. I watch it closely on the screen. I feel it in my chest. Back down to seventy-five. Sixty. Eventually it goes back down to fifty-three. Every time I go to get my device interrogated, I dread this part of the appointment.

My mom is obsessed with research on HCM. An educator, she can't help herself. With education comes research, she tells me. When I was diagnosed with Hypertrophic Cardiomyopathy she immediately conducted Google search after Google search to learn as much about the disease as she possibly could. She connected with powerful organizations like the Hypertrophic Cardiomyoapthy Association, Parent Heart Watch, and The Sudden Cardiac Arrest Foundation. These organizations all provided invaluable support.

One name kept appearing in her research: Dr. Barry Maron. Dr. Maron's name is on every study she finds. He seems to be the Michael Jordan of HCM. His medical practice is located in Minnesota. My mom calls his office and tells him our story. Dr. Maron wants to see us right away. Though we love Dr. Heller and Dr. Iyer, she decides it would be beneficial to add a specialist to the army of people keeping me safe. It can't hurt, she says.

But I can't afford to miss more school, and Dr. Maron is not covered by our insurance. We would have to pay out of pocket. My mom calls back, thanks Dr. Maron, and tells him that we won't be able to come out and see him. Dr. Maron then tells her about his son, Dr. Martin Maron, who is also an HCM specialist. He's located in Boston, at Tufts Medical Center.

My mom immediately calls Tufts to find out if insurance will cover a visit. It does! She books an appointment. I'm not thrilled to be driving all the way to Boston for yet another doctor's appointment, but I do see the value in adding a specialist to my medical team.

My parents both come with me to my first appointment, which means I'm stuck in the back seat for two hours as we drive to Boston. At Tufts Medical Center, we're directed to the Hypertrophic Cardiomyopathy Center on the sixth floor. We sit in the waiting room. I have two appointments scheduled. One is with Dr. Maron and the other is with Dr. Mark Link, an electrophysiologist.

A woman with short, dark hair opens the door to the waiting room. She looks at her file and calls out "Mike Papale." She smiles and reaches out to shake my hand. She tells me she has heard my story and that I'm a miracle. She says she's happy I'm here. This woman is Noreen Dolan. Noreen is Dr. Maron's nurse practitioner. She asks me some questions. I've heard them all before. Do you get dizzy? Do you get chest pain? Do you ever feel short of breath? No, no, and no. My mom interrupts now and then to ask a question or add a point that she thinks I've missed. It frustrates me, but I know she has my best interest in mind. She just wants me to be safe.

I like Noreen. She's very cordial, and I can tell by talking with her that she's extremely bright. She exits and says Marty will be in shortly. Marty? What doctor goes by their first name? I can't call him Marty.

Moments later, we hear a knock on the door and a tall man with dark hair walks in. He's wearing a white coat. My file is in his hand. He looks young, maybe in his thirties or early forties. He looks like he was an athlete at one time in his life, with broad shoulders. His eyes are wide. He looks at me and says, "What's up, dude?"

I'm confused. This can't be Dr. Maron. No doctor would introduce himself like that to a patient. He reaches out his hand. I go for a standard firm hand shake, but he goes for a handshake similar to one I would give Conor or John, pulling me in for a handshake-hug. A bro hug. He says, "You have a crazy story, man."

Wow. I immediately like this guy. He's cool. He's relatable. He gets me. And, when he starts talking, I immediately realize he's also brilliant. He talks about my disease. He talks about my story. He talks about what my life might look like in ten, twenty, thirty years. He has a positive outlook for my life, more positive than my own. He's confident my HCM will be treated properly. He's sure he can help keep me safe. He helps me believe that I can live a long and normal life as a Hypertrophic Cardiomyopathy patient. But, he warns, it will take time. I have to learn my body. I have to learn about the disease. I ask him questions about working out, lifting weights, shooting hoops, and more. He tells me to take it slow. He doesn't want me doing any of that yet. He wants me to take more time to recover. I don't like hearing this, but I trust him.

After spending an hour in Dr. Maron's office, we go down to the third floor to meet Dr. Link. Dr. Maron wants an electrophysiologist at Tufts to monitor my ICD. It makes sense to see both doctors during my visits. Dr. Link is a tall, thin man with silver hair and glasses. We walk into his office and, although he doesn't open up with a bro-hug, I immediately take a liking to him. He asks me questions, I ask him questions. He feels sympathetic to my family and me for all that we've been through. A nurse interrogates my ICD with the usual machine—the wand attached to the computer. I have immediate flashbacks to my first ICD interrogation. My heart starts racing, and the nurse hasn't even started the test yet. Dr. Link looks at the results and seems pleased by them. He likes the way my ICD is functioning. He likes the battery level. He looks at my scar to ensure there are no signs of infection. Everything looks great.

After a long day of appointments, we start our two hour drive back to Wallingford. I sit in the back seat feeling relieved. I start to understand the importance of a strong medical team. Dr. Heller and Dr. Iyer have been great. I trust them. I feel comfortable with them. And adding Dr. Maron and Dr. Link to my team feels like the final pieces to the puzzle. I think about one comment Dr. Maron made that day about how I can live a long and normal life. I never thought I would hear someone say that. I always thought I would be different from other people. I was unsure about my longevity. I thought my limitations would severely impact my life. I know it isn't going to be easy, but I'll do whatever it takes to live with normalcy.

SEVENTEEN

Choosing A College

My senior year of high school is flying by, so I have to determine the next step in my life journey: where I'll be attending college. I still have the list of schools that recruited me to play basketball, but they're irrelevant now. The letters have stopped coming in the mail. The phone calls to the house have ended. Those same schools that wanted me to come play basketball for them don't want me at all now that I can't play. I thought being a student-athlete is a combination of basketball and academics, but, clearly, it's just about basketball. I need a list of schools that are interested in me as a person and a student.

Conor still has his sights set on playing Division One basketball and is getting recruited by a couple of schools at that level, but he's also being recruited by many of the best Division Three academic institutions in the country. He decides to visit the University of Maine, a Division One school in the America East Conference. They're urging him to do an extra year at a local preparatory high school before coming to college and some other schools also want him to take an extra year to get bigger, faster, and stronger. The Division Three schools in the New England Small College Athletic Conference (NESCAC), however, want him to come to college right out of high school and become an important part of their team immediately. Conor is conflicted. He's laser-focused on playing Division One basketball, but knows the high-level education he can get at a lower level basketball school. He asks my opinion. I tell him to do what's going to make him happy. Life is too short to be anything but happy. I learned that the hard way.

Meanwhile, I too have to decide where to attend college and, beyond that, what to do with my life. I have a passion for my work with the American Heart Association, but I don't know if it's something I want to do forever. Maybe I can get a job working in sports. This seems fun, but I'm still unsure. Like any high school senior, I'm too young to be making such an important decision now.

I also think about location. Where do I want to go to school? Some of my friends are excited to leave home and go far away. I don't feel the same way. The thought of being far away from my family and my doctors scares me. What if something happens while I'm away? Who will take care of me? What if I go into cardiac arrest in my dorm room? I have to trust a roommate that I don't even know with my life? The thought that sudden cardiac arrest can happen at any time still gives me severe anxiety. I hate thinking about it.

My parents tell me they'll support any route I choose. I know they're scared too and want me close to home. I decide to apply only to schools in Connecticut and to commute to school. I can have fun but come home at night and feel safe. I decide I'm going to study to be a Physical Therapist. Physical Therapists can play an important role on an athletics team.

I'm accepted to Quinnipiac University, in Hamden. Quinnipiac is a gorgeous school with an incredible campus and a strong sense of community. Each building is built with brick and doesn't have a blemish. Each blade of grass in the quad is cut to perfection. It looks out to Sleeping Giant State Park, with thirty-two miles of hiking trails. It's named Sleeping Giant because of its shape. When looking at the park from the middle of Quinnipiac's campus, it's shaped like a giant sleeping on his back. I'm satisfied with my decision. Quinnipiac is the perfect place to spend the next four years of my life.

After debating the idea for months, Conor finally decides to give up his Division One dream and attend Amherst College. Amherst has an exceptional academic tradition in addition to being a Division Three basketball powerhouse. They've won multiple conference and national championships and are one of the best teams in the country every year. It's a great decision, one that will set Conor up for the rest of his life, and I'm happy for him. I wish I was going there with him, but it isn't his fault. I can't be jealous. I can't be mad he gets to do this and I don't. I know how hard he worked to get to where he is. He deserves this opportunity to make his dream come true.

I only have a couple of months left of high school. The Quinnipiac Men's Basketball team has hired a new head coach named Tom Moore. Coach Moore comes from the University of Connecticut, where he was an assistant coach for Hall of Famer Jim Calhoun. Coach Moore also served as an assistant coach on the 1999 and 2004 UConn National Championship Teams. He's recognized as one of the best high school recruiters in the country. Many of the players he recruited at UConn are enjoying successful professional basketball careers in the NBA. This is exciting news for Quinnipiac. They are just finishing construction on a brand new fifty-two-million-dollar basketball and hockey arena called The TD Bank Sports Center.

After high school graduation, I spend the summer relaxing and getting ready for college. There's no more training, no more waking up early for the gym. I still am not very active. I go on walks, but am still afraid to elevate my heart rate. The thought of my ICD mistakenly shocking me gives me the shakes. If I don't move too fast, my heart rate won't go up, and my ICD won't shock me. I hang out with my friends and spend my weekends going to the mall and the movies. I help my father prepare for another year of Hoop House Basketball Camp.

Working camp feels different this year. Some of the kids look at me funny. A lot of them were in the gym just one year ago when I suffered my cardiac arrest. They must be scared. I feel bad for them. They're so young. Some were just eight years old when they watched me collapse. A young child shouldn't have to witness such a traumatic scene.

One day my dad, some of the other counselors, and I are sitting in the gym, eating lunch. I'm having my usual: a chicken cutlet sandwich with cheddar cheese, barbecue sauce, and ranch dressing with a chocolate chip cookie from Vinny's Deli. As we watch the kids running, playing games, and having a great time, my dad has an idea. He suggests I reach out to Coach Moore at Quinnipiac to see if he'll allow me to be involved with the team. Since Coach Moore is a new coach, he might be looking for some student-managers. A student-manager? I hate the sound of this. The student-managers are the kids who aren't good enough to play and still want to be involved. Why would I want to do that? I'm good enough to play—I'm just not allowed to. But, after arguing back and forth and hearing the input from my dad and the other counselors, I give in. I'll reach out to Coach Moore.

Later that night, I put together a resume. I include a cover letter and find articles written about me before and after my sudden cardiac arrest. I want Coach Moore to know I was a player and not just a sports fan who wants to help out. The next day, before camp, I drive to the TD Bank Sports Center and drop the envelope of information off with Lori Landino, the basketball secretary. But I don't have much hope. Coach Moore is a busy guy. There's no way he's going to get in touch with me. He has a never-ending to-do list. He's hiring a coaching staff, meeting with returning players, trying to fill his available roster spots for the upcoming season, and getting settled in with his new job.

The next night, my phone rings. I don't have the number saved in my contacts, but I recognize the Connecticut area code. I pick up.

"Hello, Mike? It's Coach Moore from Quinnipiac. I received your information that you left for me. I would love to have you involved with the team. Come see me during the first week of classes and we'll talk more."

I can't believe it. This guy has won two National Championships at UConn and he's calling *me* back?

I don't know it at the time, but this is the type of person Coach Moore is. With everything else he has going on in his life, he'll take the time to reach out to an incoming freshman who wants to be involved with his program. He's a great guy.

I'm excited. This is another way for me to stay around the game I love. I think about coaching. While I sat on the bench throughout our entire high school season, it was my first opportunity to learn about basketball from a coach's perspective. If I can be on the bench at Quinnipiac, I can learn from guys who have coached at the highest level of college basketball. This seems like a great way to learn. Little do I know, this is just the beginning.

EIGHTEEN

Quinnipiac

College is fun. I meet new people and make new friends. I don't tell any of them about my cardiac arrest—I don't want them to think differently about me or to feel bad for me. I appreciate being around people who don't know my story. It's refreshing. No one asks questions. No one feels like they have to worry about me.

I need to do well in my classes. In two years I'm going to apply to the Doctorate of Physical Therapy program, which is extremely competitive. They only admit a few students each year. The program committee looks at the overall success of the student with an emphasis on their performance in science classes.

I start working with the basketball team in my free time. Coach Moore has a great staff. Sean Doherty is coming off five very successful years as the head coach at Salem State University in Massachusetts. Eric Eaton has just finished a few years as an assistant coach at the University at Albany, where he helped them win two America East championships.

Coach Moore also hires Scott Burrell, a UConn alumnus coming off a very successful playing career in the NBA, highlighted by winning the 1998 NBA Championship as a member of the Chicago Bulls. He was fortunate enough to play with arguably the greatest basketball player in NBA history, Michael Jordan.

Coach Moore also appoints Luke Murray as his Director of Basketball Operations. Luke is a young coach, just out of college, and the son of movie star Bill Murray.

I immediately take a liking to these guys. They treat me well and allow me to be involved with their work. I learn how a college basketball program operates. I'm surprised by the amount of work involved. The coaches don't just show up for practice and then go home. They spend hours in the office, meeting with players, calling recruits, and diagramming new plays. When they're not in the office they're traveling all over the country, watching potential recruits.

They let me work both in the office and on the court. One of my jobs is to send weekly letters to 250 to 300 high school prospects. The coaches also teach me how to use their video editing system so I can make film for our players to watch of themselves and our opponents. I take pride in my work as a manager, just like I did as a player.

As it turns out, I also love going to practice. The intensity reaches a level I've never seen before. Coaches are yelling, players are constantly communicating. The sound of sneakers squeaking on the floor is piercing. Everyone gets excited when a good play happens. There is no walking—the players sprint, even in between drills. They only get water when coach blows the whistle and allows them to. Even then, they only have a one-minute rest. The players are big, strong, and fast; the practices physically demanding.

I work as a rebounder and a passer. I stand on the baseline with a towel in one hand and a ball in the other. If someone dives on the floor and leaves a sweat mark, I go over and wipe it up. We don't want anyone to slip and fall. It can cause serious injury. If a ball goes out of play, I throw my ball on the court and jog off to get the errant ball so there is no interruption in practice. If a player wants to stay after practice and take extra shots, I stay after and rebound for him. Sometimes I manage the clock. Practice is scheduled down to the minute. We have to precisely utilize our time. I know every drill and how long Coach wants it to last. I keep score during scrimmages and operate the shot clock.

I love my role with the team. Everyone has a job to do, and doing your job properly is the formula to winning. I do mine as well as I possibly can. I work hard at it.

I feel my competitive fire coming back. I find I hate losing just as much as I did when I was a player, and I'm going to do whatever I can to help us win. Winning is the best feeling in the world. It solves all issues. I start talking to the coaches about their jobs and how they got them. A full-time job, coaching basketball? Forget being a Physical Therapist. When I graduate from college, I'll be a college basketball coach.

I'll do whatever it takes.

NINETEEN

Saving Lives

M y life is as hectic as ever. It feels like I have three full-time jobs. I'm a college student, I'm a student-manager for a Division One college basketball team, and I'm an advocate for heart health, CPR, and AEDs.

I start volunteering with Ryan Gomes's Hoops for Heart Health Foundation. This non-profit organization provides Automated External Defibrillators to organizations and schools that can't afford them. Ryan, an NBA player, donates AEDs on his road trips with his team, the Minnesota Timberwolves, in the different cities they play in.

Also, I find I'm not as shy in front of a group as I once was. The anxiety I used to have about public speaking has, in fact, transformed into exuberance. I enjoy talking to people about heart health. I understand the importance of telling my story. The feeling I get before speaking is similar to the feeling I used to get before playing a game. I'm nervous, but it's a good nervous, a nervous that comes with practicing and the pressure to perform well.

In the spring of my freshman year of college, Ryan invites me to be the keynote speaker at his inaugural golf tournament dinner. He expects a good crowd, but *I* don't know what to expect. My family and I pull into the Aqua Turf Club banquet facility and the parking lot is filled. There must be more than one event tonight. Nope. Everyone is here supporting Ryan and his organization. I have spoken in front of people and told my story, but never to this many people. Not even close. Men are wearing suits with ties. Women are wearing beautiful dresses. This is out of my league. Ryan greet us warmly. He's always so friendly. Everyone wants to talk to this local hero from Waterbury. He played at Wilby High School and then Providence College, where he was a First-Team All-American. He was a second-round pick in the 2005 NBA Draft by the Boston Celtics.

Ryan introduces us to Billy Donovan, the Head Men's Basketball Coach at the University of Florida, where he just won back-to-back National Championships. It is an honor to meet him. He is someone I aspire to be one day. Billy Donovan is here? For this event? And I have to get up in speak in front of *him*? I'm just getting the hang of talking in front of small crowds—I can't talk in front of hundreds of people here tonight! We sit down at our table and are surprised to find Coach Moore is here to support me. He sits with us at our table. Now I have to talk in front of the guy I look up to as a Coach and spend every day around. I can't mess this up. Dinner begins. The wait staff brings around salad, pasta, and eventually an entrée of prime rib, mashed potatoes, and vegetables. I can't eat any of it. My stomach is unsettled. I feel like I'm going to throw up. They're going to call me up to the stage at any moment. I hope I don't trip and fall. I hope I don't freeze and forget my speech.

Ryan goes onstage and takes the microphone. He talks about how he lost his friend, a former basketball teammate, to sudden cardiac arrest. It was completely unexpected. I can tell how hurt he is by this tragedy. It motivated him to start his organization, so other people don't have to lose their friends. He talks about the importance of CPR and AEDs and how everyone should be trained how to react in a cardiac emergency. He then tells everyone he's excited to introduce a young sudden cardiac arrest survivor to tell his story. That survivor is me.

I walk up to the stage carefully. I shake Ryan's hand, and he steps away from the podium. It's all mine. I have a few notes on a sheet of paper, but I want to keep my talk as natural as possible. I thank Ryan for his life saving-work. I thank him for giving people like me a chance to survive. I talk about the first time I met him, at Lido's restaurant, in Meriden. I make a joke about how he ordered the same drink, water with a lemon, as my mom, which made her day. We always gave her a hard time for her order, but now she can say an NBA player orders the same drink at dinner that she does. Then I tell my story. I talk about my cardiac arrest, how no one performed CPR right away, and how there was no AED in the building. I explain how Bob found me, agonal gasping, and the slim chances I had of surviving. I tell it all. I finish by encouraging people to spread awareness. "It doesn't end tonight. We all need to spread the importance of CPR and AEDs. The more awareness we spread, the more lives we can save. Thank you."

People start to clap. Then they stand. A standing ovation! I feel great. I shake Ryan's hand again and walk back to my table. My family is proud. Coach Moore says the speech was great. Maybe I can do this public speaking thing after all.

Later that year, the American Heart Association informs my mom and me that they want us to help lobby for a bill to get passed in Connecticut that will help save lives from sudden cardiac arrest. The bill will mandate more AEDs in public places, specifically schools. Perfect. We believe in that. The fact that a public place didn't have one a few months ago almost killed me. We both want to participate in this. We know our stories can make a big difference in whether or not this bill gets passed.

We're invited to the capitol building in Hartford and we sit in a room where legislature meets. The seats are arranged in an oval, each one with a small microphone in front of it. A group of us are going to tell our personal stories. My mom always goes before me. Sometimes it's hard to listen to her talk about my cardiac arrest. I can feel her pain. She always says, "August 24, 2006, was the most terrifying and horrifying day of my life," and, "in a heart-beat, my life changed forever." She does such an incredible job conveying her emotion while she talks that sometimes I feel like I'm the one to blame for her pain. But she's not doing it on purpose—as she talks she's having flashbacks: the phone call from my dad, the piercing sound of the ambulance, the vision of seeing me wheeled out of an ambulance on a ventilator. It's almost been a year, but for her, it feels like it's happening right now. Like me, the other mothers in the room just want to hug her tightly to help make the pain go away.

I go next. It's easy to get people's attention when you tell them you almost died at seventeen. What? How? Young athletes don't have problems with their heart. Here we go again!

Though the lobbying seems to be going well, the stories told powerful, the AHA tells us there is resistance from some legislators. They don't tell us specifically who, but they say people are worried about liability and funding to get the machines placed. I think, what's the price of saving a life? If that was *your* child out there, you wouldn't be talking about money or liability. You would want that AED to be accessible. I make sure to include this thought the next time we speak. My mom says we have to keep trying and to keep in mind that not many people have lived through what we've lived through. It isn't as clear to them as it is to us.

Over the next year and a half, we keep trying. We give more speeches. We convey more emotion—whatever it takes to get this bill passed. Finally, in 2009, we get good news: We're invited to watch Connecticut Governor Jodi Rell sign Substitute Senate Bill No. 981, Public Act No 09-94 into law! The bill makes it mandatory for all public schools to be equipped with at least one Automated External Defibrillator, for school personnel to be trained in using the AED, and for each school to set up an emergency action plan in case a student or someone on the school staff suffers a cardiac arrest.

My family and I watch as Governor Rell takes out a pen and signs the paper. Everyone applauds. We're relieved. All the hard work—the speaking, the raising awareness, and the phone calls—has paid off.

I think back to my mom coming into my room to tell me about the American Heart Association. I think about my resistance, how I didn't want to go. I didn't understand the impact we could have. Now I understand. This moment is special. This is proof we *can* make a difference. It feels better than any three-pointer I've ever made or any game I've ever won.

TWENTY

Rebuilding

F reshman year of college has flown by. I've had fun, made new friends, and found a new purpose. In the spring and summer, I help coach John's AAU basketball team. He's playing for the Central Connecticut Hoop Stars, a program my dad created when I was younger. I grew up playing in the program, with Dad as my coach. Now John is playing for our dad, who allows me to join the team as an assistant coach. My basketball knowledge is expanding after my first year observing the Quinnipiac coaching staff.

I help our team understand how hard they have to work in practice to perform well in the games. I watched hard work in practice translate to wins in my first year as a student-manager.

It's a fun summer. I spend a lot of time with my family, traveling throughout the Northeast to compete in different tournaments, just like we did when *I* was playing. And I love coaching John. It's fascinating to see him evolve as a basketball player and as a person. I know if he keeps working hard he has a chance to be a very good player.

Before I know it, classes start up in the fall. I'm done with Physical Therapy—I don't need to be a Physical Therapist to coach college basketball—and I start taking Media Studies classes. They're interesting and also a way to stay involved with sports as a broadcaster or journalist if I don't end up coaching.

Meanwhile, I continue to visit my medical team and pass my check-ups with flying colors. My heart muscle isn't getting thicker, I still feel no symptoms and my ICD battery is still very high. The scar is completely healed, and there are no signs of infection. All is good. Except one thing – the weight gain. I still haven't lost any of the weight I put on after my cardiac arrest. I'm 225 pounds, thirty-five more pounds than I weighed before I stopped playing basketball.

As a nineteen-year-old college student, I still don't understand the importance of having a good diet. I still want to eat whatever I want to eat. The guys on the team don't have strict diets, and they're in great shape. Of course, they burn thousands of calories every day at practice, but I don't think about that.

Bottom line: I'm still afraid to work out. I don't want to go into sudden cardiac arrest again. The thought of running and getting my heart rate up causes me to panic. Dr. Heller and Dr. Maron try their best to assure me that my ICD will save my life if something happens. That's the purpose of me having it. But I don't want to get to that point. I don't want the ICD to have to save me.

The other students look like they're in good shape. The players are all confident walking around the arena with their shirts off. This is hard for me. My confidence is low. I don't tell anyone, but I hate my body. I feel hopeless, like this is never going to change. This is how I'm going to look for the rest of my life. Losing confidence has a huge impact on my life.

I want to get back down to under 200 pounds, but to do that I need to make a lifestyle change. If I don't, 225 can be become 250, or even more, and lead to other health issues. The more weight I gain, the harder it is on my heart. I need to regain control of my body. I have to practice a better diet and get over my fear of working out.

Dr. Heller suggests I sign up for cardiac rehabilitation. There's a program in Meriden that she can get me enrolled in. I reluctantly agree. She thinks this is the first step for me to learn how to work out safely and confidently.

Cardiac rehabilitation consists of three phases, with each patient's participation based on their individual situation. Phase one begins in the hospital. Patients are educated on cardiovascular risk factors and the signs and symptoms of a heart attack or sudden cardiac arrest. Patients are given at-home exercise guidelines, consisting mostly of walking. In phase two, patients exercise in a cardiac rehabilitation department while nurses monitor how the patient responds. The patients are watched closely at all times on a telemetry monitor. Phase three includes workouts that are supervised by nurses but with no telemetry monitor. Phase one lasts from one day after admission to the hospital until hospital discharge. Phases two and three can last anywhere from four weeks to one year, depending on the patient's individual situation. I'm placed directly into phase three because of my age and current health condition.

I go to my first session and immediately hate it. I don't want to be here. The guy on my left looks like he's eighty years old. The guy on my right is definitely in his sixties. I'm nineteen, the youngest person in the room by at least fifty years.

The nurses tell me to get on the treadmill. I've done this before. I don't mind running on a treadmill. We start, and the speed is four. It's a slow walk. I walked faster when I came into the building. This must be my warm-up. Nope. They don't let me go any faster.

Next is dumbbell curls. I like this. It's time to work on my biceps. The nurse tells me to grab the set of blue dumbbells in the corner. I walk over to get them. Five pounds? I ask, "Are you sure these are the right dumb bells?" The nurse is positive. I think, what is the point of *this*?

The program lasts four weeks. Eventually, the nurses let me do a light jog on the treadmill and eventually a steady run. They allow me to lift heavier weights. My heart rate increases. I start to sweat. But my ICD doesn't shock me. I feel great. I can safely work out. I'm not at the finish line yet, but cardiac rehabilitation is the start I need to get control of my lifestyle.

After graduation from cardiac rehabilitation, I start working out daily on my own. I go to the YMCA, just like I used to with Conor. But, instead of playing basketball, I spend my time in the weight room. I use the cardio machines. I lift weights. I stretch. I pop my head in the gym to see if anyone is playing basketball. I can't play, but if a hoop is open I'll take some jump shots before heading home.

I'm confident I can safely push my limits when I exercise. It's not nearly the level of intensity I once trained at, but it's better than doing nothing. The more I work out, I'm finding, the more comfortable I become.

The next step is to change my diet. This isn't so easy. When traveling with the team at Quinnipiac, we order food every couple of hours. We have food for us on the bus when we leave for a road trip. We get to the hotel late at night and there's more food. We wake up in the morning and there's a breakfast buffet, followed by chicken parmesan for a pre-game meal. After the game, on the bus, is a post game meal. I have to be disciplined. I can't eat what everyone else eats if I want to lose weight. I eat more salads. I eat fewer carbohydrates. I decline the late-night food at the hotel. I only eat dessert for special occasions and completely cut soda out of my diet. I know I'm not eating the perfect diet, but I'm eating a better one.

Soon I notice a difference. The hard work is paying off. When I look in the mirror in the morning, I don't want to close my eyes. I step on the scale and the number is back down below 200. I also notice my life improving. I have more energy. I'm more excited to wake up every morning and start my day. I feel confident about my appearance. I'm not afraid to take my shirt off in front of other people. I feel myself getting back to the old me.

TWENTY-ONE

Refocusing My Goals

A s I learn more and more about the college coaching industry, I decide that, when I graduate, my goal is to get a full-time job with a Division One basketball program. This won't be easy. There are only 347 Division One basketball programs in the country. If I want to get a job, I know I have to separate myself from the many other candidates. My resumé isn't going to say "former college basketball player" or "former professional basketball player." It's going to say "former student-manager," and that makes the task even more difficult. A lot of former collegiate and professional players transition into coaching when they retire. I flash back to the day my dad told me I needed to separate myself as a player if I wanted to play in college. I did that. I need to have the same mindset with coaching. I need to work harder. If I don't, someone out there is working harder than I am. Everything I do must bring me one step closer to reaching my goal. And the first step is to give everything I have to Quinnipiac Basketball.

Any time I'm not in class or studying, I'm at the basketball offices working with the coaches. As soon as class ends, I get in my red, two-door Pontiac and drive one mile down the road to the TD Bank Sports Center. I ensure the coaches see me there at least once every day. I'm determined they see how hard I work to help make their program successful. I always present myself properly and professionally.

My ultimate target is to become a Director of Basketball Operations. Most Division One programs offer this entry-level position. Usually, young coaches hold the position for a few years before they move on to an assistant coaching role. I want Coach Moore to think he has to hire *me* when his Director of Basketball Operations position opens. I want to earn his trust over the four years I'm there and make sure he knows he cannot hire anyone else.

As the days go by, I work harder and harder. I stay late in the office with the coaching staff to watch game films. I help the assistant coaches with their scouting reports. I handle all of our team meals when we're on the road, making sure they run smoothly and quickly so we're in and out of restaurants to maximize the players' rest the night before a game. In the summer, I help direct the Tom Moore Basketball Camp, which runs for two weeks every year, using my experience at Hoop House Basketball Camp.

I treat every single day of my four years at Quinnipiac as a job interview for the Director of Basketball Operations position.

TWENTY-TWO

John's Basketball Dream

Half-way through college, another summer approaches, which means another summer of AAU basketball. This year I'm the assistant coach again for John's team. My dad is still the head coach, but he gives me more responsibilities with the team. I'm getting more experience coaching and using the knowledge learned from my dad and from my time at Quinnipiac.

It still hurts not to play. All those weekends in a gym and I can't help but wonder if I'll ever fully get over the fact that I can't play basketball. I miss it. Sometimes, watching other kids have fun playing makes me sad and jealous. But I also feel lucky that I can still be around it. Watching John helps fill that void. I find myself living vicariously through him.

John has completed his sophomore year at Sheehan High School, where he had a lot of success on the court. He was brought up to the Varsity team as a freshman and played a lot of minutes. As a sophomore, he played only Varsity, but in a reserve role: He didn't start, even though he might have been the most talented player on the team. John never complained. He just did the job that was assigned to him. I know being a reserve bothered him. It bothered me. I think he deserved to start. Even as a reserve, he finished his sophomore year as one of the team's leading scorers.

After his sophomore season, John is recruited by the head coach at Choate Rosemary Hall, Adam Finkelstein. I'm excited for him. People are noticing how he's developing as a player and as a person.

Choate is one of the most renowned academic preparatory high schools in the entire world and is located in our hometown. It boasts an incredible alumni list, including President John F. Kennedy, presidential nominee Adlai Stevenson, actor Michael Douglas, and many more. Choate offers an opportunity to change his world completely.

Choate has a higher tuition than many universities. It attracts students from all around the world. Luckily, we live in town and John can live at home, thus avoiding the cost of room and board. He applies and is accepted, and I can tell how excited he is by the ear to ear smile on his face. He isn't very emotional, but he knows this can have an incredibly positive impact on his life. Choate gives our family a financial aid package my parents cannot pass up.

John will be attending Choate as a repeat sophomore, giving him an opportunity to get adjusted to the course load, which is much more demanding than at Sheehan. It will also give him an extra year of high school basketball to get him ready to play in college. Coach Finkelstein tells John he's going to push him hard. He's going to bring everything out of him so he reaches his full potential both on and off the court. This is the perfect situation for John, who has the same dream I had: to be a college basketball player. He's on the right track, and with three more years of high school, he's going to be in the perfect position to make this dream come true. I *want* his dream to come true. I *need* it to come true.

TWENTY-THREE

Battling For March Madness

I head into junior year feeling more confident than ever. I'm consistently working out and eating a much cleaner diet. I've lost all of the weight I gained after my cardiac arrest, and my doctors are happy with the progress I'm making. My ICD battery is still high. The thickening of my heart hasn't changed. Most importantly, I know what I want in the next phase of my life: I want to coach college basketball.

We have a great team at Quinnipiac this year. Our senior and junior classes are both very talented. We cruise through the regular season, finishing with an overall record of twenty-three wins and ten losses and a conference record of fifteen and three. Two of our players make the All-Conference Team. Our eyes are set on the conference tournament. If we win, we'll earn a spot in the NCAA Tournament, the ultimate goal for a Division 1 Mid-Major school. Quinnipiac has never played in the NCAA Tournament, and we want to be the first team to take them there. We're the number one ranked team in the conference, so if we keep winning we'll host all the conference tournament games, giving us a big home court advantage.

In the first round we play Monmouth University, from West Long Branch, NJ. We split with them during the regular season: They beat us on their home court, but we beat them when they came to our gym. The regular season doesn't matter anymore. It's now one and done: If we lose one game, it's all over.

We feel the pressure in the first half of the game. Our players look nervous and hesitant on the floor. They don't seem themselves. We head into halftime down two points, 33 to 31. Coach Moore ignites our team at halftime with a powerful speech. We belong here. We were the best team all season long. It's time to show everyone that. We score fifty-three points in the second half, win the game 84 to 75, and advance to the semi-finals.

In the semi-finals we face, Long Island University from Brooklyn, NY. We only played them once during the regular season and won. When the game starts we look like a different team. Our nerves our gone. We look like the team that dominated throughout the regular season. We jump out to a 39-32 halftime lead and never look back. We win the game 83-78. One game away from winning the conference championship, the NCAA Tournament is in our sights. The team in front of us is Robert Morris, our archrivals. Robert Morris beat us and knocked us out of the conference tournament semi-finals last year. They didn't only beat us, they won by twenty-seven points. It was embarrassing. We want revenge. The good news: we played Robert Morris once during the regular season this year and won.

Campus is buzzing with excitement about the game. Everyone knows this is Quinnipiac's chance to make it to the NCAA Tournament for the first time in school history.

We have two practices in between the semi-final and final games. Our players watch film carefully, they practice the scouting report, and they work on their shooting. They spend extra time in the athletic training room, ensuring their bodies are feeling good and ready to perform at the highest level in the championship game. We have the team shoot around the morning before the game for one hour. Everyone is laser-focused. There is nervous energy, but also feelings of extreme excitement. We finish our game day preparations with a team pre-game meal. Everyone is ready for tip-off.

Quinnipiac's colors are blue and gold. Our athletic director wants the whole arena to shine in gold that night. The plan is to pass out gold t-shirts to every person who walks through the doors. Tip-off is in ninety minutes. I'm doing my usual pre-game work, which consists of making sure the film equipment is set up properly, organizing the bench, and rebounding for our players as they get ready to play. The gym is still empty. No fans are allowed in yet. When the clock hits sixty minutes, we go into the weight room with our team to stretch while the doors open and fans start to enter the arena.

We come back onto the court after fifteen minutes, stretched and ready to go. My jaw drops. The seats are filled with gold. With forty-five minutes on the clock the arena is completely filled. And people are *still* coming in. Where are they going to sit? The gym starts to get hot. People are screaming. The horn goes off and the game is about to start.

Our arena seats about 3,500 people, but there has to be 5,000 people in the gym right now, most in gold and rooting for Quinnipiac. There's a group of fans in blue behind the Robert Morris bench, a small army of supporters that took the trip from Pittsburgh, PA. Up in the concourse people are standing three rows deep. I'm thankful I'm sitting right behind the bench. I look up into the stands again. My parents are at the game, in their usual seats. They come to all of John's and my games. If there is a game going on, at least one of them is there.

The starting lineups are announced and people are screaming and cheering, but during the National Anthem you can hear a pin drop. The air is thick with tension. We're moments away from both teams fighting, desperately, for a championship. The players walk onto the court. The referees blow the whistle, and the ball is thrown up into the air. Finally, the game has begun.

Both teams are nervous. This is the biggest game most of these players have ever played in. It will take some time to break the nerves. The first basket isn't scored until one minute and forty-five seconds have run off the clock. Finally, the ice is broken. Ten minutes into the game the score is even at ten. Both teams are playing as hard as they possibly can. The coaches are doing the same. They're coaching their hearts out. With less than a minute to play in the first half, we lead 25-21. Robert Morris has the ball. They make a shot, cutting our lead to two. We have the ball with one more chance to score before halftime, but we miss a three-point shot attempt. At halftime, the scoreboard reads Quinnipiac 25, Robert Morris 23.

I feel good at halftime. I think we're the better team. We deserve to win this game. Our guys are playing hard, and they're going to play even better in the second half. The crowd is on our side tonight. It feels like no one in the arena has moved. Everyone is standing still. They don't want to miss one second of the action. In his half-time speech Coach Moore reminds our players how hard they've worked to get here. We belong here.

After fifteen minutes we go back out onto the court.

Twenty minutes on the clock separate us from our first ever Northeast Conference Tournament Championship.

The second half is a battle. No team leads by more than four points. With ten minutes to go in the game, we're ahead 38-36. The action continues to go back and forth. We lead by one, Robert Morris leads by two, we regain a one-point lead, and Robert Morris takes it from us to go up by two again.

Suddenly, there's a minute left. How? It feels like we were just in shoot-around earlier this morning and now we're one minute away from determining the championship. We trail 50-48. My stomach hurts. I'm nervous. I want to win this game more than any game I've ever played in.

We have the ball and have an open shot, but out of nowhere one of their players flies in to block it. Where did he even come from? It's an incredible play. There are only ten seconds left, and we're still down by two. We have to foul and send them to the free throw line and hope they miss. But they make both free throws to go up by four. We come down quickly and score, cutting the deficit to two with just five seconds left. We foul again, and they miss both free throws. We get the rebound, down by two with four seconds on the clock. We immediately call timeout.

This is it. One play. We have one final shot to tie or win the game and keep our hopes alive. Coach Moore draws up a play on his whiteboard. The players watch intently. Everyone is nervous, even though they're trying not to show it. The horn sounds, and the players walk back onto the floor. The referee hands our player the ball. We throw it in bounds to one of our guards. He takes four dribbles and heaves up a three-point shot. We all stand. If it goes in, we win. If it doesn't, we lose. Everyone's eyes are staring at the ball. It's moving so slow, I can see the laces on the basketball spinning perfectly.

It falls short. The buzzer sounds. We lose. Robert Morris celebrates on our home floor. We walk back into the locker room, crying, devastated.

I have been a part of many losses in my life, and it's never easy. Losing is emotional, but it happens. No one wins every single game they play. The emotion in this locker room, though, is unlike anything I've ever seen before. Players are sitting on their chairs with their heads tucked into their laps, weeping uncontrollably. They can't stop. The coaches' eyes are red as they try to hold back tears. An entire season of hard work came down to this game, and we lost. I'm crying too. I thought this was our year. I thought we were going to the NCAA Tournament. I didn't play, and I'm not a coach, but losing hurts just as much for me as it does for them.

I wonder if we'll ever have another opportunity to make it back to the championship game. I hope so. I hope this wasn't our only chance.

TWENTY-FOUR

Head Coach Papale

My dad has a new job with Metro North as a conductor on the railroad. He'll no longer be able to coach John's AAU team, but he thinks I'm ready to take over the job. I'm excited, and I think I'm ready, but I've never been a head coach before. Here's my first chance to take everything I've learned from my time as a player, a student-manager, and coaching with my dad to create my own coaching philosophies.

But I also have to think about my heart health. There is added pressure being a head coach. You're standing on the sidelines the whole game. During tight games, will my heart rate go up? Will being a head coach affect my blood pressure? I talk to my medical team about my thoughts and they give me the okay to give it a try. After all, I do have an ICD that will shock me if it needs to.

The season starts in the spring, after our season at Quinnipiac ends. We have practice two times per week. I love being able to run the practice as the head coach. I'm able to mold the team as I see fit. We travel to different

AAU Tournaments throughout the Northeast on the weekends.

But I notice my relationship with John starting to crumble. It's a struggle for me to balance being his brother *and* his head coach. I'm harder on him than anyone else. I yell at him more. I don't mean to do it, but it just happens. I'm more passionate about how he plays than the other kids on the team. We argue and fight during practices and games, which isn't good for the other kids to see. We don't hang out as much anymore off the basketball court. He seems sick of me. I realize I have to change my actions.

John is doing all of the right things and is now getting recruited by multiple Division One schools. He's working hard and playing well. I have to learn how to communicate better with him. After a couple of tournaments, I back off. I start treating him like I treat the other kids. I don't scream at him during the games if he isn't playing well. I talk to him. I try to coach him. Our relationship begins to reform.

I'm learning on the fly as well. As a first-time head coach, I have to learn how to plan practices with limited gym space, manage a team of nine kids, give them each the playing time they deserve, and showcase our players in front of college coaches. I have to learn how to coach a game, manage timeouts, and adjust in the moment. I'm trying to discover my own coaching style.

Our last tournament of the season is AAU Nationals at Disney's Wide World of Sports Complex in Orlando at the end of July. The best AAU teams in the country will be participating. There will also be college coaches present to recruit our kids to play in college. I remember when I was out there, playing and fighting for a spot on a college team. It's now my job to help my players get recruited.

The tournament starts with a pool play format. Each

team is placed in a pool with three other teams. The top two teams from each pool advance to the championship bracket. We play well and win all three of our pool play games, finishing in first place and advancing. College coaches are following our team closely, especially John. He usually has ten to fifteen coaches at every game watching him play.

The championship bracket begins, and we start slow in our first game. We're not playing well at all. We look tired and nervous. We're playing another team from the Northeast called the CMA All-Stars. We get down by fifteen points early in the game. It doesn't feel like we have the will to come back and win. I call a timeout. I bring the kids in and try to get them excited, but they look defeated. I tell them we still have a chance if we turn it around right now. The scorekeeper blows the horn. The timeout is over. I ignore it. I keep talking to the guys, telling each and every one of them to go out there and fight for their lives. The referee comes over and tells me to bring the kids back on the floor. I ignore him. I give a few last words. The referee is now annoyed that I'm ignoring him, but I don't care. It's more important that I get our team ready to start a comeback. He blows the whistle again as we're coming out of the huddle. My energy is high, my emotions are flowing. I flip my white board up in the air in frustration and let is smash on the ground behind the bench. The referee blows his whistle again. He gives me a technical foul for unsportsmanlike conduct. This is the last thing we need. We're already losing. The other team now gets two free throws and the ball back. But somehow the timeout and technical foul sparks our team. The guys are remotivated and ready to fight. We make a ferocious comeback to win the game.

We win our next two games and advance to the quarterfinals of the tournament. It's another tight game. The team we're facing is good, but I think we're better. Our team plays well early, and we lead by six at halftime. We start the second half slow, and the game is tied up. It goes back and forth. With twenty seconds remaining, we have the ball and the game is still tied. We're letting the clock run down before we take a shot to win. With ten seconds on the clock, one of our players drives the ball to the hoop. He gets fouled and is awarded two free throws. I think we have the game won. All he has to do is make these two free shots. The first one is in the air, hits the rim, and falls out. Now he looks nervous. He shoots the second one, and it has no chance. It falls short and hits the front of the rim. The other team gets the rebound, throws the ball down the court, and makes a miracle shot to beat us. It's another devastating loss, and I feel like I'm responsible for it. We should have held onto the ball longer so the other team didn't have the opportunity to make the miracle shot. I call the team together and tell them we have to forget about the loss. We don't have time to be sad. We have more games to play starting tomorrow.

We play three more games and win them all, finishing in fifth place, the best finish by a team from our program. Our fifth-place trophy is huge and heavy. We all take turns signing the basketball on the trophy with a sharpie. It's a great ending to my first year as a head coach.

I learn a lot that season about coaching. I learn coaching is much more than just basketball. Yes, my job is to help our players improve individually, and help our team improve as the season goes on to win the most games possible, but it's also my job to serve as a mentor and role model for our players throughout the season. I'm only four years older than most of them, but I want to provide a good example of how to act both during competition and off the court when we travel. I ensure that the kids know they can come talk to me if they have any issues, even if the issues aren't basketball related. I want them to feel comfortable coming to me to talk if they have an issue at home or in school. Being a coach is about helping kids grow, mature, and get ready for the next phase of their life, both on and off the basketball court.

TWENTY-FIVE

Quinnipiac Senior Year

P rior to my senior year, we find out that Quinnipiac is funding our team to go to Europe to play four games before school begins. We will play in The Netherlands, Belgium, and France. This is my first opportunity to travel outside of the United States, and it's completely paid for. I'm thankful to Quinnipiac. Without them, I wouldn't have this cultural experience.

Our first stop is The Netherlands. From LaGuardia Airport it's an eight-hour plane ride with a layover. I have never been on a plane this long before. I'm in and out of sleep for most of the ride, and when we land at our final destination, I have no idea what time it is. The Netherlands is six hours ahead of us. I feel exhausted. We get off the plane, grab our luggage, and meet our tour guide. He tells us we can't go to sleep—we have to stay awake to beat the jetlag. We get on a bus and head to our hotel in Amsterdam. We're just dropping off our luggage before we get back on the bus to do some sight-seeing. He takes us to the Anne Frank House. As we walk through the house I think about the courage this woman had. Her life feels surreal to me. I thought I had troubles with my medical condition but her struggles make me feel like I had it easy. As we walk around the city, I notice there are bikes everywhere. Not only are people riding them, but thousands of bikes are locked on racks on the streets. If you don't look as you walk across the street, you might get hit by a bike. We try stoopwafel and herring, two popular local foods. The portions are small. We're hungry shortly after we eat, so we find another café. At night, we walk downtown. It's very different than anything we've ever experienced. Club promoters are standing outside trying to convince us to come in. We spend three nights in Amsterdam, play and win one game, and get on a bus to head to Belgium.

We take the games seriously—the kids play hard, and Coach Moore coaches hard—but once the game ends, Coach ensures we spend as much time as possible exploring these countries. This is more about the experience than about the games.

As we cross into Bruges, where we will be staying, I feel like I'm in the center of a painting in an art gallery. The Neo-Gothic brick style is breathtaking. Each building is carefully crafted with a unique structure and design. After checking into a Marriott directly on one of the canals, we start to explore. There are more bikes—not as many as as in Amsterdam, but still enough to make it seem like this is the primary mode of transportation here. The city is filled with canals and bridges. We head down to the market and see Belfry of Bruges, a medieval bell tower on Market Square. We see the beautiful churches and eat the famous chocolate. We win another game, and head to France.

We're staying in Paris, an eight-hour drive. The city looks very familiar. It reminds me of New York City, with huge buildings and a lot of people. There are cafés at every corner, famous for their baguettes and croissants.

We explore Musée du Louvre, home of the *Mona Lisa*. We also see the Cathédral Notre-Dame de Paris and Avenue des Champs-Élysées. Our final tourist destination is the Eifel Tower. There is a long line, but we wait it out. We finally get to the front, and they put us on an elevator. The floor is glass, so we can see the ground, which isn't a big deal until we start going up. The ground is getting farther and farther away from us. I'm not afraid of heights, but I don't want to look down. Still, I can't help myself, so I look. The ground is so far away, I can barely see it. At the top the view is amazing. We can see for miles. We explore Gustave Eiffel's office and look at the panoramic maps to see how far we are from major world cities. The wind is blowing, but since we're so high up the noise from the city disappears. After spending thirty minutes snapping pictures and admiring the views, we head back down. We play two games in France, winning both easily. Then we head back to the United States.

We land a few days before classes begin. It's time for me to start zeroing in on my future plans. I know I want to coach at Quinnipiac, but if there isn't a job open for me, I'm going to have to look elsewhere. Even if there is a job open, there's no guarantee Coach Moore is going to hire me.

I ask to meet with him for advice. He respects how hard I've worked for the program and suggests I start reaching out to every college program in the Northeast by sending them my resumé and a cover letter expressing my interest in coaching at their school. It doesn't matter if they have a job opening or not. Even if they don't, this is a great way to network.

I get right to work, creating packets of information, similar to the one I submitted to Coach Moore four years ago. I send them all out, hoping to get a response from someone interested in hiring me.

At Qinnipiac we're looking forward to the upcoming season. We need to avenge our loss to Robert Morris. They've eliminated us from the tournament two years in a row. One of our seniors, Justin Rutty, who won Most Valuable Player in our conference the previous year, is ready to have a stellar senior year, win the award again, and carry our team to the NCAA Tournament. With him on the team, we have a chance to actually win it all this year. We have another strong regular season.

We finish the season with an overall record of twenty-two wins, eight losses, and a conference record of thirteen wins and five losses. Justin has a good year, but he's not as consistent as he was his junior year. He has nagging injuries holding him back, on and off, throughout the season. But we're back in the Northeast Conference Tournament, and again we need to win three games to win a championship. We're hosting Mount Saint Mary's from Emmitsburg, MD, in our first game. We played them twice during the regular season, with each team winning one game. This time we get off to a fast start and go into half-time with a 41-34 lead. Our team is ready. We're experienced—we've been here before.

We dominate the second half and win the game 78-59. Next on the schedule is none other than Robert Morris, standing between us and another chance at playing in the Northeast Conference championship game. Everyone on the entire campus wants to beat Robert Morris. We haven't been able to get past them, and we're tired of losing.

We get another good crowd for the game. The arena is almost sold out. Forty minutes for another opportunity to reach the Northeast Conference title. We know it's going to be another battle.

A back and forth first half ends with us leading 33-29. We have to sustain the lead, but we start slow coming out of halftime, unable to score for the first three and a half minutes. Robert Morris takes a four-point lead and seizes control of the game. We battle back to tie the game up at fifty-one. No team leads by more than two points until there are two minutes left on the clock, when Robert Morris has a four-point lead. We make a three-pointer, cutting the lead to just one point. We're right there, again. We play good defense, and they don't score. We have the ball now, with a chance to take the lead. One of our players is fouled. He makes two free throws. We lead by one.

Robert Morris comes down the floor after calling time-out. Now one of *their* players is fouled. He makes the first free throw. Tie game. He misses the second. All we have to do is grab the rebound, but Robert Morris steals it from us. They have the ball. The game is tied with forty seconds on the clock. They call a timeout to diagram a play. All we needed was one rebound, and we didn't get it.

They come out of the timeout and their point guard dribbles in place as the clock ticks down from forty, thirty, twenty seconds remain. He starts to make his move. Our players are right in front of him. He drives to the rim and throws up a shot.

We play great defense—no way this can go in. The ball hangs in the air and drops through the net.

Six seconds remain, and we trail by two. We call a timeout. It feels like we're in the same situation we were in just a year ago. Down two to Robert Morris on our home floor. We need one basket to tie or win the game. Coach Moore draws up his play. The players listen intently. I hate this feeling. It's way too familiar.

We come out of the timeout and inbound the ball. We

drive it quickly down the court and take a three-pointer. The ball falls short. We lose to Robert Morris again.

It's heartbreaking. The locker room is reminiscent of last year, with a lot of tears. Our seniors come to the realization that their college basketball playing career is over, a harsh reality for so many athletes. And my career as a student-manager is over. I've given four years of dedication to this program—four years of hard work, four years of trying to make it to the NCAA Tournament. Now it's over. It's time to move on. It's time to start my own coaching career.

Meanwhile, John is in the middle of an important high school season. He's a junior and hitting his full potential. Choate wins the Class A New England Preparatory School Athletic Council Championship, and he's named Most Valuable Player of the tournament. College coaches are at every game. And these are not Division Two or Three coaches recruiting him—they know John is too good to play for them. The only schools coming now are Division One. He's considered one of the best three-point shooters in the entire country.

May arrives and I graduate from Quinnipiac with a Bachelor of Arts in Media Studies. During our graduation ceremony, I reflect on my college career. Our commencement speaker is Mitch Albom, author of the inspirational book _Tuesdays with Morrie_. He's also a sports journalist, screenwriter, broadcaster, and musician.

I think about how far I've come in four years. I realize how crucial these years were for me: I recovered from my cardiac arrest, both physically and mentally; I met some great people; I had an experience working with a basketball team that has set me up to launch my coaching career. I enjoy the rest of the ceremony and the celebration that follows, but tomorrow I have to get back to work. I have to find a job. Nothing has worked out yet, but that doesn't mean it's time to quit. It means it's time to work harder. I need to keep networking.

John has one more summer of AAU basketball to play before his senior year of high school. He decides to leave my father's program. He's out-grown it as a player and needs something bigger where he will get more exposure. He gets recruited to play for an ADIDAS sponsored team called the New England Playaz. The Playaz are one of the top AAU teams in the country, with many former players now at the highest level of college basketball and even playing professionally. They're coached by former Duquesne University and Boston Celtics coach John Carroll, who gives me the opportunity to be an assistant coach on the team. This is just what I need. I get to spend the summer with John and also network with other coaches in hopes of finding a job.

We spend the summer traveling all over the country. This team doesn't just compete in the Northeast like our old team did. We compete at tournaments in New Jersey, Connecticut, Rhode Island, Massachusetts, Arkansas, Oregon, Indiana, Minnesota, Nevada, and California throughout the spring and summer. Coaches from the most prestigious basketball schools in the country are watching our team play against some of the best players in the country, some of whom will go on to play in the NBA in a couple of years. John has a great summer. He plays very well. He attracts attention from Division One schools all over the country and finishes with full scholarship offers from more than thirty schools.

Now he has to narrow his list. He's not going to sacrifice a great education just for basketball. He wants to find a perfect mix of both academics and athletics. He narrows his list to Harvard University, Boston University, Fairfield

University, University of Vermont, Northeastern University, College of the Holy Cross, and Towson University. John has spent hours on the phone communicating with these coaches. The next step in the recruiting process is to take visits. He has to see which school is a good fit for him. We spend much of August visiting different campuses. John likes the schools he visits, but he never seems blown away. So far, he hasn't found the perfect place for him, but we still have two more campuses to visit.

In late August, we plan a one-day visit to see Boston University in the morning and Northeastern University in the afternoon. John has always loved Boston, and I have a good feeling that he'll end up at a school there. We drive up to Boston and find our way to the Boston University campus, where the head coach, Joe Jones, has just gotten the job. He was previously the top assistant at Boston College and spent time as the Head Coach at Columbia University, as well as being the top assistant at Villanova University. Coach Jones is full of energy and clearly excited to see us. He's about six feet-one in a bright red Boston University polo with black shorts. When we arrive, he gives us all a big hug. He has a lot of energy and an infectious personality. His assistant coaches are also a great group of guys. They drive us around campus and through the city. Later, we sit in a conference room while Coach Jones presents some information about the school. He talks about his vision for the basketball program and how John will fit in. He talks about the high-level education John will be getting if he attends BU. Everything sounds great. We go to the student center and have lunch. We talk to the coaches about their pasts and what attracted them to BU. We also walk through the basketball arena, the weight room, the locker room, and the film room. The coaches take us to one of the dorms called Student Village, which is two separate towers where juniors and seniors live. They bring us up to the top floor, where we look out the window and see the Charles River, and behind it, the whole city. It's a beautiful summer day, not a cloud in the sky. Out of the corner of my eye, I see John smile. He looks happy. The combination of a great basketball program, top academics, nice facilities, and a view like this is perfect. I have a feeling John is going to commit to play basketball at Boston University.

We get back in the car and head to Northeastern, right down the road. As we drive down Commonwealth Avenue, the weather starts to change. Dark clouds appear in the sky. It gets windy. As we park our car and get ready to go inside, it starts to downpour. There is thunder, lightning, and heavy rain. The coach meets us outside with umbrellas. We take the visit and enjoy it. Another great academic school with great basketball tradition, another great opportunity for John. The coaching staff is friendly and welcoming to all of us. As we listen to the coach make his pitch, I'm thinking John has his mind made up, but he listens respectfully.

The next morning, John calls Coach Jones. He accepts a full scholarship to play basketball at Boston University. His dream has come true. He's going to play college basketball.

TWENTY-SIX

College Coach

I have two job interviews. The letters I sent out have finally paid off when two coaches call to say they have a position available. Southern Connecticut State University and the University of Massachusetts Lowell. Both schools compete in the high-level Division Two Northeast-10 Conference. I'm not sure what to expect in these interviews, but they go well and lead to two job offers.

I think about which job is the best fit for me. I want my first job to continue my development as a young coach and a young adult. And it's time for me to move away from home. I'm ready to do this. I'm healthy and confident living with my heart disease. I call Greg Herenda, the head coach, and accept a position as an Assistant Basketball Coach at the University of Massachusetts, Lowell. I'm twenty-two years old, just out of college, and ready to take everything I've learned and bring it to Massachusetts.

UMass Lowell is a great place to start my coaching career. I get to do a little bit of everything. I'm recruiting potential student-athletes, writing scouting reports about our opponents, and working out the players to help their individual improvement.

Coach Herenda is intense. He demands excellence from both his players and his coaching staff, including me. He pushes me to be a better coach. I haven't been pushed this hard since I stopped playing. I'm not a manager anymore—I'm a coach, and I have to act like one. He teaches me how to get the most out of our players in both practices and in games. I learn the strategies behind his offensive and defensive schemes. He teaches me about his responsibilities as the leader of the program, knowing my goal is to one day be a head coach. As intense as Coach Herenda is on the court, *off* the court he's fun to be around. He invites me to his house and lets me spend time with his family. He cooks me dinner. He pushes me to get better, but always has my best interest in mind.

We have another assistant coach on staff by the name of Marc Kuntz. He's the top assistant and has been coaching in college for close to ten years now. Marc teaches me the ins and outs of being an assistant: how to talk to recruits, what to look for when watching film, and what to focus on when writing my scouting reports. He gives me drills I can use to help with player development. Marc and I share an office and spend a lot of time together each day. He becomes a close friend and someone I rely on throughout the year.

We have an exhibition game against Providence College before our first regular season game against the University of Bridgeport. The night before we play Providence, Bridgeport is playing in an exhibition game against Fairfield University. My job is to drive down to scout the game and then drive back to Lowell for the game against Providence the next day.

I drive down to Fairfield University, which is thirty minutes from home. My dad and John meet me there. I take as many notes as I can on Bridgeport's team. I don't want to mess up my first scouting report. After the game I drive back up to Lowell, feeling excited. We're playing Providence tomorrow. My first game as a coach is against a Big East team. I'm not ready to go to bed yet, so as I drive, I call one of my friends, an athletic trainer at UMass Lowell. I ask him if he wants to go out for a drink. He agrees, so I pick him up and we go to a couple of our favorite bars in downtown Lowell. We hang out for a couple of hours hour before I drop him off at his apartment and head home. I pull up to my house around 1:30. It's late and I'm ready for bed. I want to get some rest before the big game tomorrow. There are two guys walking down the road as I pass by. They're walking in the same direction I'm driving, and I wonder what they're doing walking around so late.

I pop my trunk and get out of my car. I have a case of water I want to bring in the house. Suddenly the two guys run across the street toward me. This can't be good. Adrenaline is shooting through my body, yet I can't move. It feels like my feet are in cement. The guys approach me. One stands inches from me. He's wearing a mask. He yells, "Give me your stuff!" I turn around. Another guy in a mask. This one is holding a gun, and it's pointed right at my head.

I say, "It's all yours." I immediately throw my phone, my wallet, and my keys on the ground. They grab my belongings and run away. They run about fifty feet and then turn around. They yell something at me and throw my keys back in my direction. I let them run away so far that I can't see them before I grab my keys and quickly go inside, wake up my roommate, an assistant coach on the women's basketball staff, and use her phone to call 9-1-1. Seven police cars show up within minutes, their lights flashing, lighting up the neighborhood. They advise my roommate and me to move from this area. The officer says it's starting to become infested with gang violence. Thankfully, the two men didn't hurt me.

I finally get into bed. It's past 3:00, and I have to wake up early. I need to rest but I don't sleep. I can't. I stay up for the rest of the night in shock. I think about the man pulling the trigger. I've already almost died once. If he'd fired the gun, the police would have found me lying on the sidewalk in a pool of my own blood. If the men hadn't liked my reaction, they could have killed me and run away. I try not to think about it. I think about the big game tomorrow.

We leave for Providence College early in the morning on a coach bus. It feels like a dream walking into the Dunkin Donuts Center, a 12,200-seat arena. I'm standing on the floor, helping our guys warm up, running on adrenaline with no sleep from the night before. The buzzer sounds and the game is about to begin. My first game as a college coach. Here we go.

We aren't supposed to win the game. Providence is a high-level Division One team, and we're Division Two. In fact, they're paying us money to play the game and whoop our butts. It's a tune up game for their regular season, a chance for their fans to see them win an easy game. But Coach Herenda doesn't allow our team to buy into this. He makes our team believe we're going to win the game. We're going to surprise everyone. We're going to leave Providence with a nice check for the program *and* a victory.

The game is going back and forth—too close for comfort for Providence. They maintain a small lead but we're right on their heels. With just eight seconds on the clock, we have the ball. We're down just one point. We call timeout, and Coach Herenda draws up a play for our best player to take a shot. The play works—our players execute it to perfection—and the shot goes up. The ball rattles in . . . and then falls out. We lose by one. What a game! Our team is upset—we just had a chance to take down a Division One team—but we're optimistic about the upcoming season and the success we can have.

We have the next day off from practice, so I go home to get a new license, a new wallet, a new phone, and a new debit card—everything that was stolen from me. I go back to Lowell on Sunday night but never sleep in that same house again. My roommate and I decide we need to find a new place to live. I crash on some different coworkers' couches before we find an apartment in Nashua, NH, about fifteen minutes from campus.

Throughout the season I listen closely to Coach Herenda and Marc. I take their criticism. They're teaching me to be better at my craft. We finish with a record of nineteen wins, eleven losses, and go to the conference championship game, where we lose to Stonehill College.

As the year ends, I decide I want to try to get a Division One job. UMass Lowell has been a great step in the right direction, but I want to move up. I really want to go back to Quinnipiac and work for my alma mater, but there are still no jobs open there. I have to look elsewhere. If nothing else works out, I'll go back to UMass Lowell for a second year.

Early that September, I'm sitting on my couch when I get a call from one of the assistant coaches at Quinnipiac. Their Director of Basketball Operations position just opened up. Jon Iati, their current Director of Basketball

Operations, has just accepted a job as an assistant coach at the University at Albany.

I immediately update my resume and send it to Lori, the basketball secretary, who hand-delivers it to Coach Moore's desk for me. Coach Moore calls me later that day. He invites me to come in for an interview next week.

TWENTY-SEVEN

The Dream Job

It's a beautiful fall day in September as I'm driving to Connecticut from Lowell. The leaves are changing and the foliage is breathtaking. I've been waiting for this moment since I started working as a student-manager: an opportunity to be a full-time member of a Division One college basketball coaching staff is finally here.

I want to go in to my interview prepared. I spend the night creating a portfolio for Coach Moore. He needs to see how badly I want this job. I buy a nice three-ring binder and fill it with a long, detailed resumé of everything I accomplished in my one year at UMass Lowell. Coach Moore knows me as a student-manager, but I want him to know what I can accomplish as a coach. He's interviewing one other guy who played for him at Quinnipiac, and I need to separate myself from the other candidate. I spend the night rehearsing possible answers to questions I think he might ask. When I finally go to bed, I know when I wake up the next morning I'll be ready.

I drive to the TD Bank Sports Center for my interview. The drive is so familiar, having done it every day for four years. I can basically do it with my eyes closed. I listen to the song "One Shining Moment," by David Barrett. This song is played every year after the National Championship game on CBS, with a montage of highlights from the entire tournament. It feels like this is my one shining moment.

During my four years as a student-manager, I worked tirelessly to prove my worth. I walk into the arena directly to Coach Moore's office, knowing in my bones that I deserve this job.

The meeting turns out to be more like a conversation than an interview. Coach and I have known each other for four years. He knows my personality. He asks about my family and how everything is going with my heart condition. He asks me about my experience coaching at UMass Lowell and how that experience has helped my development as a coach. I tell him I've been preparing for this job for years. I can start tomorrow without any assistance or training. I'm ready to go. I show him my portfolio. He looks through it, carefully dissecting the work I did the previous year. After talking for an hour, we stand up and shake hands. He says he'll call me next week and let me know his decision.

I walk out of the interview feeling nervous. I think I nailed it, but I don't know what Coach Moore is thinking. Maybe he wants to stay loyal to his former player. Maybe he doesn't think I'm the best fit for his staff right now. Only time will tell.

I drive back up to Lowell to continue working for Coach Herenda. I hate the waiting game. I just want to know one way or another about the job. I pester the other assistant coaches at Quinnipiac daily, hunting for feedback from the boss. They all think he's leaning toward hiring me, but my nerves persist.

A few days later, while watching a Boston Red Sox game with some friends, my phone rings. The caller ID announces Coach Moore. This is the moment I've been waiting for. I step outside to take the call, a quick walk, but a million thoughts shoot through my brain. This conversation is either going to be really positive or really negative for me.

I answer. Coach Moore asks how I'm doing and how my family is doing. I appreciate his kindness, but want him to get to the point. He says how hard of a decision he had to make. He knows I already have a great coaching job, so he'd thought about giving the other guy a shot. My heart starts to drop. Then he changes his tone. He says he knows I'm the perfect fit for his staff. He knows I'll be able to step in right away, and he offers me the job!

I'm ecstatic. This is literally my dream coming true. He tells me I can think about it if I want to, but I know I don't need to. I accept the job on the spot. I know Quinnipiac is where I want to be and where I want to continue my collegiate coaching career.

I work at UMass Lowell for another week, finishing up my responsibilities for Coach Herenda and the rest of the athletic department. I reflect on everything I've learned throughout the year and how appreciative I am for the opportunity Coach Herenda has given me. He gave me my first college coaching job. He made my college coaching dream come true. And Coach Herenda knows this is a good move for me, he knows how special it will be for me to coach at my alma mater. I leave on good terms with him and Marc. I complete all of my obligations with them in Lowell by the end of September before moving back to Connecticut to start my new job early in October.

My first season as a coach at Quinnipiac is up and down for us. We have a good, young team but just can't piece together a bunch of wins in a row. We win a couple of games and then lose a couple games.

I circle one important game on my calendar: Sunday, December 16, 2012, the day we're playing against Boston University, John's team. He has just been inserted into the starting lineup and is playing well as a freshman. We're both ultra-competitive, and we both want to win this game badly. It puts my parents in an awkward position, and our mom wishes the game will end in a tie.

The game comes down to the wire. We're up by three with ten seconds remaining. I think we're going to win. They have the ball and need to go the full length of the court to score. During the timeout I wonder who will get the last shot. It can't be John. He's only a freshman. John inbounds the ball to his roommate, also a freshman and the starting point guard on the team. He dribbles the ball up the court quickly, and John stays behind him. John cuts hard to his left, then quickly back to his right. He's about thirty feet from the basket when his roommate flips the ball back to him. John takes the shot. The ball looks like it's on a good line . . . right through the hoop. My kid brother hits the game-tying shot at the buzzer to send the game into overtime, during which John scores eight more points, including two three-pointers to help win the game for BU.

This is awkward. Everyone on our team knows we're brothers. I never want to lose to him, but I do want him to succeed. I just push him in the hand shake line, and we laugh. He has bragging rights for the next year.

At Quinnipiac, we finish the season losing in the semi-finals of the conference tournament. We have a lot of young players and are ready to come back stronger next year.

TWENTY-EIGHT

Career Goals

My schedule is chaotic. Coaching takes up a lot of my time. During the season we're traveling every week, staying in hotels. In the offseason, I'm in the office for hours preparing schedules, workouts, and film for our players. But I can't complain. After all, my job is basketball. One down side: I don't have as much time to volunteer with the American Heart Association anymore. I attend the occasional event or heart walk when I can, but that's it.

Before the 2013-14 season, we find out we're changing conferences. We're going from the Northeast Conference to the Metro Atlantic Athletic Conference (MAAC). This is a huge upgrade for the university and the athletic department. The MAAC is a vastly better and more competitive conference. We have a lot of players returning from the previous year and add some key recruits, positioning ourselves to have a strong showing in our first year in the new conference.

BU is on the schedule again in December, but this time on Quinnipiac turf. I'm eager to get revenge on my brother and win back the Christmas dinner table bragging rights for the year. It's a huge game in our local community. John is arguably the most successful basketball player our town has ever seen, and he's returning to play against his brother's team. We both have very good teams this year, so we know it will be a good game.

The game is a close one and tied as the clock winds down. They have the ball for the final possession, and one of John's teammates makes a shot just as the buzzer sounds. They beat us for the second year in a row. John still has the bragging rights!

Although we lose that game, we have a very successful season, surprising a lot of people during our inaugural year in the MAAC. We go to the conference semifinals, which nobody expects us to do in our first year.

I'm happy about my life. My dream job at Quinnipiac is going well. My health continues to stay steady. I check in with Dr. Maron and Dr. Link, and everything is looking good. My ICD battery is getting lower—which means I'll need surgery soon—but not until the summer. I feel good. I'm staying active, working out daily. I feel confident about living my life with HCM. Dr. Maron told me the day he met me I can live a normal life, and now I finally feel like I am.

I think about my future and the next step in my career. I can't be a Director of Basketball Operations forever. I have to continue to work to advance, so I spend my time, again, trying to prove to Coach Moore that I'm ready to be an assistant coach.

TWENTY-NINE

A Routine Surgery

n August 2014, after my second year as Director of Basketball Operations at Quinnipiac, it's time for me to get the battery of my defibrillator replaced for the first time. I want to get the surgery done before the new basketball season begins—I don't want to miss any time with the team.

I'm confident about the surgery. I don't feel nervous about it. I've been through it a few times and know the drill. After all, this is a routine procedure. The doctors simply have to open the pocket where the battery is placed on the upper left side of my chest, detach the battery from the wires, and replace it with a new battery. While in surgery, the doctors will manually put my body into cardiac arrest to test the device.

My mom and I drive to Boston for the outpatient surgery. My dad is planning to meet me at the hospital in the recovery room.

During the procedure, the doctors remove the old battery and place the new one. Now they have to test the device. The device could recognize the life threatening rhythms, but it didn't have enough energy to terminate them. They try again and have the same issue. The device isn't giving enough power to shock my heart back to a normal rhythm.

When I wake up I'm dazed and confused. Dr. Link tells me the news. I immediately flash back to being seventeen years old, finding out the first surgery was unsuccessful. Frustration sets in. I wonder if the device would have actually saved me if it was needed in the previous eight years. I'm glad I didn't have to find out. Another setback.

Dr. Link gives me two options. Option one is to add a third wire on the left side of my chest to add more power going directly into my heart. Option two is to try changing my medicine, because they think it might be controlling my heart rate and blood pressure so much that the device cannot pick up an irregular rhythm. This is the same decision we had to make eight years ago.

I talk it over with Dr. Link and Dr. Maron and compare the options with my family. We decide it's best to have the third wire surgically implanted the next day. I'm not comfortable switching my medication at this point. My body has adjusted to it. I've been taking it for eight years and haven't had a problem.

I still don't feel nervous for the next surgery. I've learned to maintain a positive attitude and am confident with my medical team. I know they'll keep me safe.

I go in for the surgery, and, sure enough, Dr. Link successfully places the third wire. They test the device, and it works perfectly. After recovering for one more night in the hospital, I go home.

Thankfully, this surgery doesn't require a long recovery. My left arm is stiff, but other than that I feel normal. I have a lot of energy and can go to work immediately. But I take some time off from working out because it takes a couple of weeks to regain a full range of motion in my left arm and shoulder.

I'm excited about my third season as the Director of Basketball Operations at Quinnipiac. I'm fully recovered by the time our players return to campus in September and we have another good team coming back for our second year in the MAAC.

THIRTY

Complications

P ractice starts and the guys appear hungry to have a great season. One day, after practice, I go to New Haven for dinner and drinks with some of my coworkers. We're sitting at the bar enjoying ourselves when my chest starts to itch. It's itchy on the spot where my ICD is located. This has never happened before. I don't think it's anything serious—I'm sure it's nothing—but the itch won't go away.

I drive home and get ready for bed and, as I'm changing, I look in the mirror. My chest is red and swollen right on my ICD. It must be irritated from me constantly rubbing the area. I go to bed thinking it'll be gone when I wake up, but the next morning nothing has changed. It still itches and is still red. Still, I drive to the office, thinking it will go away.

Usually, I don't even think about my ICD, but today is different. Today, it's all I can think about. The itchiness doesn't stop. I can't stop touching it, and nothing makes the feeling go away. I call my mom to see what she thinks. She is always overly cautious, more so than I am. She tells me I should call Dr. Link immediately and let him know. I try to avoid calling my doctors unless it's completely necessary, but I think this is a good reason. I've had an ICD for eight years and this has never happened to me before. I call Dr. Link and his reaction surprises me—he says he needs to see me tomorrow. He has never rushed me in for an appointment. He thinks the device could be infected.

I drive to Boston early the next morning. Dr. Link examines the irritation, which is not as bad as he expected it to be. He prescribes a strong antibiotic medication that will help reduce the swelling as quickly as possible. I take the medication for ten days as directed, and the itchiness, the redness, and the swelling go away.

But after a few days go by something still doesn't feel right. My neck is stiff, and my body feels worn down-- constantly. I tire more quickly than normal and need to go to bed earlier. Finally, a few weeks later, in mid-November, after our second game of the season, I decide to drive back up to Tufts and see if something else is going on. Dr. Link doesn't think my stiff neck and my other side effects are being caused by an issue with the defibrillator, so I keep moving forward, hoping these issues will go away.

The next week, I have one of the longest night's sleeps I've ever had in my entire life. One minute I feel extremely hot and start sweating profusely, the next I'm shivering cold and grabbing extra blankets. I can't get comfortable. It's excruciating. I feel like I'm getting sick—really sick. It must be a twenty-four-hour virus. I'm sure it will go away within a day. I wake up in the morning and go into work. I still have a fever. I feel awful. I take Tylenol, which helps, but as soon as the medication wears off, I start shivering and sweating again. I fight through it.

Walking through the hallways back to my office after practice, I pass by Alyssa Budkofsky, our team academic advisor and one of my close friends. Alyssa is among the most respected members of our program. She works tirelessly to ensure our players are successful during their four years in college. She mentors them, hosts study halls, makes sure they're keeping up with their assignments, and, most importantly, takes the role of acting as a mother for everyone in the program.

She stops me in my tracks. My teeth are chattering because I'm so cold. She tells me I don't look good and that I need to go home. I hate being sick. If I go home, I'm letting the team down. But Alyssa persists. I back down and go home, thinking one more night of sleep and I'll be healed.

I wake up the next morning and, to my disappointment, I'm wrong. In fact, the virus seems to be getting worse. My body is aching, and my temperature is spiking at 103.

Our team is traveling to Albany that night to stay in a hotel before a game against the University at Albany tomorrow. I have to be there with the team. In the meantime, my mom decides to take matters into her own hands. She calls Dr. Link and tells him about the extreme fever, and he knows something is terribly wrong. Now, positive my device is infected, he calls and orders me to be at Tufts before the end of the day. I try to convince him that I'm getting better. I lie and say the fever is going down. If I go to Tufts, I can't travel with team. This is the last thing I want to happen right now. We hang up the phone without reaching an agreement. I tell him I'm going to give it a couple more hours and see how I feel. Minutes after we hang up, my phone rings. It's Dr. Link again. He tells me I have two options. I can get in the car with my mom, and she can drive me up to Tufts, or, if I continue to refuse, he will be sending an ambulance with sirens on to pick me up.

I realize he's serious. I concede and tell my mom I'll drive up with her.

I still think I'm going to somehow travel with the team. I don't know how, but I'm going to make it work. I inform my mom that we'll be driving straight from Tufts to Albany that night. I text Coach Moore to keep him in the loop. I tell him I'm coming on the trip, but I have to first go to Tufts to be examined. Coach tells me I need to go to the hospital and not to worry about the trip at all, my health is most important.

As I sit in the passenger seat of my mom's car, I'm miserable. The car ride is agonizing. My body cannot regulate itself. I'm freezing, so I put on multiple layers to warm my body, but after sitting in the car for just twenty minutes, my body is now hot and I can't stop sweating. I take all the layers off. Minutes later, it's back to being cold. The Tylenol isn't working at all anymore. The sweats and the chills keep coming back the entire ride.

Later that night, John is playing in one of the most exciting games of his collegiate career against the undefeated and top-ranked team in the country, the University of Kentucky. Kentucky is loaded with NBA talent. They have so much talent, in fact, that they sub five players in and five players out every few minutes. The talent level doesn't drop even when their reserve players enter the game. They are that good. The game is being played in Rupp Arena, which holds 23,000 screaming Kentucky fans. They're the favorites to win the National Championship and haven't lost a game yet this year. My dad flew out to Kentucky to support John. As we drive, I keep a close eye on the time. The game tips at 7:00 p.m. I have to watch it, the biggest game of John's career.

We arrive at the hospital a little after 7:00, just as the game is starting. I'm still extremely uncomfortable, shifting back and forth from freezing cold to extremely hot, but I pick up the live stream of John's game on my phone. We walk to the cardiac floor, where I'm given a room. They tell me I'll be staying overnight. I won't be making it to Albany after all. The first question I ask is how to log on to the Wi-Fi so I can watch John's game on my lap top. The game ends around 9:00, and John's team loses, as expected. But it's surreal watching my brother play against the best team in the country. I call my dad after the game and ask to talk to John. I tell him how great it was to watch him play. I tell him I have to stay in the hospital overnight, but I'm fine. John knows something is off. I don't sound like myself. He doesn't say anything, but he's glad I'm in Boston so he can visit me when the team returns. It's Friday, November 21, 2014, six days before Thanksgiving. I assure him I'll be going home before the end of the weekend, and I'll be back in Boston to pick him up so he can come home to celebrate Thanksgiving.

Conor and I have a Thanksgiving tradition. We go out to the local bars on Thanksgiving Eve to meet people we grew up with. John is usually not able to participate because his basketball schedule is too grueling. But this is the first year he's been given a couple of days off. It's the first time the three of us will be able to celebrate this tradition together.

Conor is now living in Los Angeles, working for BNY Wealth Management. He's flying into Boston Wednesday morning; the same day John is scheduled to go home. We have a plan in place. I'll drive to Boston on Wednesday to pick up Conor at the airport, then we'll go pick up John at school and head back to Connecticut.

I'm convinced we'll still be able to execute the plan. There is no way I'll be stuck at the hospital past the weekend. I call Conor, letting him know my situation, but not to worry. I'll be there at the airport Wednesday morning to pick him up.

A nurse comes in and tells me they need to take blood to determine what's causing the extreme fevers. I've had plenty of blood taken in my life. I don't like it, but not a big deal. She then tells me she cannot give me any more medication to control the fever. They need to take the blood when I'm experiencing one of my freezing cold or extremely hot states. I must let them know immediately so they can come in and draw the blood. I don't sleep for one minute that night. I try, but I can't. I'm miserable. The night feels like it's never going to end. They get the blood sample they need. The fever keeps hitting, making my body shake.

THIRTY-ONE

Infected

My body has never done this to me. Why is it happening? The sun starts to rise and I'm desperate for answers.

Dr. Link and the Tufts MC's infectious disease team diagnose a staph infection that has settled onto the metal components of my implanted defibrillator. They tell me my body has no way to fight it. They start pumping me with antibiotics to keep the infection at bay. If they don't move quickly, there is a possibility the infection can spread to my blood stream, which would be imminently life threatening.

After discussing different possible options, Dr. Link decides my ICD has to come out to eradicate the infection from my body. They have to remove the battery, and, using a carefully focused laser, extract the wires as well. There's a possibility the infection has traveled to the wires, which are directly touching my heart muscle.

This is the last news I want to hear. I thought the bad news was all in the past. Also, this is an intensive surgery and comes with further potential complications. But there is no other choice. My life depends on it.

Dr. Link explains the risks. There's a chance that, while the surgeon is extracting the wires with the laser, the scar tissue surrounding the wires will rip and cause bleeding in my heart. If I lose too much blood, I can die in surgery. This is going to be more intense than any surgery I've ever been through.

Just in case I started bleeding, an additional surgeon will be on hand, Dr. Warner, a specialist who will perform emergency open-heart surgery to save my life. The doctors and nurses assure me there is only a one to two percent chance of this happening. They have experienced multiple lead extractions before and the need for open heart surgery is very rare. I convince myself it won't happen.

I'm scheduled to go in for the surgery on Tuesday, November 25, 2014, the night before I planned to pick up John and Conor in Boston. Our Thanksgiving plans are now cancelled.

The night before any surgery is always a long one. I've been through this before, so I'm used to it. I spend the night mentally preparing myself, forcing myself to believe everything is going to go smoothly. I have the TV on again, trying to keep my mind busy. *The Fresh Prince of Bel-Air* has now been replaced by the HBO series *Entourage* as my favorite show. I've seen every episode and can recite them in my head. I finally doze off, ready to get the surgery behind me.

I wake up the next morning and, after all that waiting, Dr. Link informs me that my surgery has to be postponed until the next day. Someone in the hospital needs an emergency heart transplant.

I'm disappointed. Another day of waiting. This doesn't seem fair. I want to get this over with. But I also think of the person who needs an emergency heart transplant and gain some perspective. This person is having their heart completely taken out of their body and replaced with a completely different heart. My surgery isn't going to be routine, but I know it won't even begin to compare to the intensity of a heart transplant. It makes me realize that, as difficult as my situation is, I have much to be grateful for. There are people out there experiencing worse.

THIRTY-TWO

Thanksgiving Eve

The surgery is rescheduled for the day before Thanksgiving. My mom, my dad, and John come to the hospital to support me as the medics prepare me for surgery. I feel calm and relaxed. We sit in a waiting room while they place IVs into my arms, just in case open heart surgery is necessary. But everything will be okay. At a young age my mom taught me to say, "I'm strong, I'm healthy, I'm in control." This mind trick has never felt more necessary. I recite it over and over again in my head until I truly believe it.

I give my family a hug, and the nurse wheels me down to the operating room. It's cold, just like I remember it. The surgery is set to begin at 1:00 p.m. and will last about four hours, though the doctors did caution my family it can take longer if they have to perform the emergency open heart surgery. As I slowly drift off to the anesthesia, with the nurses and doctors surrounding me, I feel at peace. I start counting. 1 . . . 2 . . . 3 . . . out.

My family sits in the waiting room eagerly waiting for

the surgery to end. They have been in this situation before too. Seconds feel like hours and minutes feel like days.

Hours pass, and there is no word from the doctor. The waiting room is silent. Out of pure nervousness, nobody says a word. My family sits there waiting…and waiting…and waiting.

"Something's wrong," says my mom, whose sixth sense tends to hit high alert when it comes to the well-being of John and me. Seconds later, her phone rings. It's Dr. Link. Finally, some news.

But it isn't news anyone wants to hear. During the removal of the right atrial lead, Dr. Link explains, there was a perforation. As they were extracting one of the leads, the scar tissue around it started bleeding, and Dr. Warner had to perform emergency open-heart surgery to save my life. My family is told my blood pressure keeps dropping to a dangerous level, and there is a chance I might suffer serious brain damage. My mom bursts into tears and exits the room.

"This is way too much," she thinks, as she paces Tufts MC's halls. "To have to live through not one time almost losing my son, but a *second* time…is unbearable." With great effort, she calms herself and returns to the waiting room, feeling sure her reaction has scared everyone. She reminds herself she has no control over the situation. There is nothing to do but wait.

Not knowing how long this will last, John goes back to his dorm to try to sleep while my parents wait for me to get out of surgery. They can't leave until they see me.

Hours later, Dr. Warner returns to explain that my body has gone through a serious trauma and has required *eight* blood transfusions. There is still concern about serious brain damage. He says only time will tell.

As he speaks to my parents, the sound of a stampede fills the hallway, getting louder each millisecond. And then: eight medics speed by, surrounding a gurney and heading toward the recovery room. Someone is holding a ventilator on the patient. The patient is me.

THIRTY-THREE

Back To Intensive Care

I spend the rest of the night unconscious on a ventilator. My condition is finally stable. As the morning comes, the anesthesia starts to wear off. I become alert, and my mom asks me if I'm okay. The ventilator is still in, so I can't speak, but I try to smile and give her a thumb-up sign.

I'm confused. No one has told me about the complications yet. I have a catheter in, as well as multiple IV's. One IV is going into the vein in my neck. I can feel a big bandage over it. I can't move my head. My body feels stiff and sore. The walls ahead of me are painted a tan color and are completely blank besides a clock that reads 8:00.

I immediately think the surgery went well. I went in earlier that afternoon. The surgery must have gone for a few hours. After recovering and the anesthesia wearing off, it makes sense that it's 8:00 p.m. The nurse tells me to take a long, deep breath. She slowly takes the ventilator out of my throat. It hurts. I hate the feeling. I finally am able to look around and get my bearings. I turn to my right and there's a window. The sun is up. It's bright outside. It can't be 8:00 p.m. The sun sets before 8:00 p.m. in November. I realize it's 8:00 a.m. the next morning. Something went wrong. The surgery was not supposed to take all night.

With my throat still sore from the ventilator I ask the nurses about the surgery. The nurse explains the complications and emergency open heart surgery. I'm shocked. I can't believe what she's telling me. It feels like the rest of the anesthesia wears off instantly. I feel very alert now. They tell me I'm in the Cardio Thoracic Intensive Care Unit (CTICU).

I look at my parents in disbelief. We have already gone through so much with my medical issues. They have had to endure so many waiting rooms and surgeries that have lasted longer than expected. I feel bad for them. They are just happy to talk with me. It is a relief after the conversation they had with Dr. Link just a few hours ago.

I hate being in the CTICU. Everything is being monitored. All I hear is beeping coming from the medical machines in my room. I have flashbacks to my horrible memories spent at Connecticut Children's Medical Center in their intensive care unit. I have four tubes sewn into my stomach to help drain the blood and fluid oozing from around the surgical site. These tubes keep the blood and fluid from accumulating in my chest and compressing my heart or lungs. My chest is really sore. A few hours ago, they performed a sternotomy prior to starting the open-heart surgery. Sternotomy, or the opening of the sternum, is another word for cracking the sternum and opening up the rib cage. Every time I cough, sneeze, laugh, or move the wrong way, I'm in severe pain. I have a red pillow shaped like a heart next to my bed. It's there to put over my chest to ease the pain. I feel like I've been run over by a bus. I've been through many surgeries and many recoveries, but none have made me feel like this.

I beg the nurses and doctors to get me out of the CTICU and put me back on a general cardiac floor. I don't mind the regular floor. I had my own private room when I was there. I feel more relaxed in that environment. I don't think I can handle being in the CTICU for an extended stay. I ask the medical team what needs to happen before I can move. They tell me I need to be able walk without assistance. Once I can walk, I can go to the general cardiac floor. This seems simple. I'm determined to get out of bed and walk right away. I try but can barely stand up. I finally get myself out of bed, but I'm holding onto the bed rail to keep myself from falling over. I try to take a step. It hurts. I can't move. I feel like I'm going to fall on my face. My parents watch and cringe as I struggle. I look at them and I feel like my world is shattering.

THIRTY-FOUR

Progress

A couple of days go by. I don't even try to get out of bed, but I can finally sit up on my own. Eventually I'm able to get out of bed and move over to a reclining chair. Anything is better than lying in bed all day. I start walking very slowly and with the help of others. Doctors monitor my progress and inform my parents they don't think I have suffered any brain damage after all. This is a huge relief. Soon I'm able to move back to the general cardiac floor.

For the first time in eight years I do not have an ICD in my body. I touch the place on the left side of my chest under my collar bone where my ICD used to be. There isn't a bump anymore. It's flat. I wonder when I'll have a new ICD put back in? I know it's crucial to my longevity. If I don't have one, I won't be able to keep living the normal life I've worked eight years to create for myself.

Dr. Link says I need to recover from the open-heart surgery before anything is done. They continually check the amount of blood draining from my body each day. All patients bleed in the early hours after open heart surgery.

The amount of drainage varies by patient. They chart my weight loss and monitor my appetite. Most importantly, it's crucial my body is clear of the staph infection. They pump my body with antibiotics through the IV multiple times each day.

The recovery is slow and frustrating. I wish I could fast forward time. I want to count the days until I can go home, but the medical team doesn't know when they'll be able to discharge me.

A couple of days go by and I'm able to start moving around more and more. I can walk on my own. No one has to hold me up. But it feels like I'm moving at a snail's pace. Dr. Warner comes in and tells me he's going to remove two of the tubes that are sewn into my stomach. This is good news. A step in the right direction. He has me lie flat on my back in the bed so he can examine me. He tells me to take a deep breath in and hold it. I follow his direction. He then tells me to slowly exhale. As I exhale, he rips the tubes out. For a second, I can't breathe. It feels like I've been sucker punched in the gut. I look at him thinking there has to be another way to get these tubes out. There isn't. I'm finally able to catch my breath, and Dr. Warner says he'll be back tomorrow morning to remove the other tubes. I hope tomorrow morning never comes. I don't want that feeling again.

I stay up all night, dreading the next morning. I feel anxious. *Entourage* is playing in the background but I'm not focusing on that. The only thing on my mind is having the remaining tubes removed.

Dr. Warner arrives bright and early. I haven't slept. I feel tired. This is the last thing I want to happen right now. At least this will be over in a few minutes, and I'll never have to think about it again. He examines the tubes. He says they need to stay in one more day. Great. Another sleepless night. Another night of lying here and thinking about getting the wind knocked out of me in the morning.

The next morning, he removes them. The experience is the same. I hold my breath and he just rips them out. I lose my breath. I hate the feeling but the tubes are gone.

Visitors come every day to check on me. I feel lucky. It helps the days go by faster. My parents and John are always there. This is a hard time for all of us. Dr. Maron isn't officially treating me, but he comes to my room occasionally just to check on me.

Meanwhile, John is in the middle of his basketball season. He's a junior captain for the team. He goes to practice every day, travels for games, goes to class, studies, and in between everything, he comes to see me. We don't talk much about these tough times. We talk about anything else. But we're both there for each other. Seeing him and hearing about his practices and games are the highlight of my day. We've both been here before, but instead of being seventeen and thirteen, we're twenty-five and twenty-one.

I continue to get stronger. I'm walking more and my appetite is improving. I'm also sleeping a lot. Dr. Link is confident we can move on to the next phase of my recovery, which means I can go home soon. The ultimate goal is to have a new ICD placed, but the doctors first need to be sure the infection has completely exited my system. If they place the ICD too early, the infection can settle back on the device, and we'll have to start over.

He tells me a peripherally inserted central catheter, or PICC line, is going to be placed in my right arm. He's willing to let me go home, but I have to continue to administer antibiotics when I leave. The PICC line will be similar to the IV, so I can give myself my antibiotics each night.

Two nurses come into my room to place the PICC line. They numb my right arm so I won't feel anything. The plan is to place the PICC line through a small hole just above my right bicep. It doesn't hurt, but the sensation is odd. It feels like a worm is crawling up my arm, under my skin, from my bicep to my shoulder. I close my eyes. I can't wait for them to finish. Suddenly, the nurses act confused. They keep asking each other questions. Neither nurse has an answer. Something isn't right. I sit there silently, frightened, waiting for them to tell me they're done working.

When they finally stop, they tell me the installation didn't go as planned. It's not placed properly. They have to come back another time and try again. Frustration and anger shoot through my body. I can't go home until this PICC line is placed properly. How could they possibly mess this up? My parents come in the room, but I don't want to talk. They leave me alone, and I wait.

The next day, the nurses take me downstairs, where a specialist will look at the PICC line to see if it can be fixed. They want to try this instead of removing it and placing a new one. I lie on my back, and they numb my arm. After thirty minutes, the PICC line is finally in the correct place.

Since I don't have an ICD in my body, Dr. Link gives me a Zoll Life Vest to take home with me. This is my ICD until the new one is placed. It will save my life if I go into cardiac arrest. He teaches me how to wear the life vest properly. It has wires attached to it that will constantly read my heart rhythm. I have to wear it under my clothes with the leads directly on my bare skin. I have to wear it at all times, except when I'm in the shower. It will start beeping if the leads are not on properly and the vest is not able to read my rhythms. There is a chance the machine can mistake a good rhythm for a bad one. They teach me how to stop the machine from shocking me if it makes a mistake. If I'm conscious and hear the noise indicating a shock is coming, and physically able to, I can stop the unnecessary shock from happening. This sounds scary, but there's nothing I can do. If I want to go home, I have to wear the vest. I'm not arguing with anything they say. I don't want to delay my departure from the hospital another minute.

Dr. Link wants to monitor me for one more night to make sure there are no more setbacks. If everything looks okay in the morning, he'll send me home.

Another night with no sleep. Another long night of thinking. What if the open-heart surgery didn't go well? What if I did have brain damage? What would that even be like? I can't imagine a life without being able to remember anything. I think about my current condition. I've lost a lot of weight and blood. My body feels much weaker. My sternum is still broken. I also think about the future. When can I work out again? When can I get back to practice with the team? Will I be able to get back to normal after another setback? I know I have a battle ahead, but by the end of the night I feel ready to face it.

THIRTY-FIVE

Homeward Bound

After fourteen days in the hospital, it's time to leave. I'm sitting in the chair in my hospital room, and a nurse comes in and takes out the IV. I feel free. Dr. Link says I'm discharged and can go home. I wait for the wheelchair to show up. No wheelchair. They let me walk to the car.

My parents and I start the two-hour drive back home to Wallingford with very mixed emotions. I'm feeling relief to get out of the hospital, but I'm still nervous. I know I have a long battle ahead. It's going to be challenging, but I have to be patient. The PICC line will be in for six weeks. My parents are overwhelmed. The last two weeks were completely unexpected and a whirlwind. We all hope my recovery will be as smooth as possible.

After five minutes, as we turn right to get on the Massachusetts Turnpike, my Life Vest starts beeping. We panic. I'm worried the device is going to shock me. I don't know what to do. It's under layers of clothing, including a winter jacket, so I won't be able to get to it in time before it shocks me. My dad quickly pulls over, puts the car in park, and jumps out. The beeping is constant. I unbuckle my seatbelt and quickly take off my jacket. I pull off my shirt so I can see the leads. One has come off my chest. Thankfully, it's nothing serious. The device is just informing me the lead isn't properly placed. I fix the problem, and we continue our trip home.

Waiting for us in Wallingford is a home nurse whose job is to train us how to properly use the PICC line pump. The nurse is an older man who seems to be irritated. He's very sarcastic and, at this point, none of us have the energy to deal with his sarcasm. We just want to learn how to use the pump so we can all get the rest we desperately need.

The PICC line is sticking out of my arm. The area where it's placed is covered with bandages and wraps. I have to attach a battery-operated automatic pump to the PICC line, and each night I install a new medicine bag to the pump. Each bag lasts one full day. The pump is small enough that I can hold it in my hand if I want, but too big to fit in my pocket. The kitchen counter is filled with medical supplies, making it look like a hospital cabinet. There are bags of medicine, alcohol wipes, and pain medication.

For the first couple of days, Dr. Link wants me to rest, so I sit on the couch, read, and watch TV. The open-heart surgery stole so much energy from me, I keep falling asleep. Every time I go for a walk, I tire within minutes. Also, the PICC line and life vest are annoying. Everywhere I go I carry a backpack with the battery for my life vest and the pump for medication.

Just changing my shirt is a long process, because each time I do it, I have to detach the pump from the PICC line. I wrap my arm in towels and plastic every time I shower so the PICC line doesn't get wet. Everything is a struggle and takes longer than necessary.

Luckily, visitors continue to come in and check on me. Everyone is in shock when they see me. I don't look like myself. I've lost at least fifteen pounds and look skinny and frail. No one can believe how tired I am.

One day, I just need to get out of the house, so I attend a basketball practice at Quinnipiac, where I'm greeted with a warm welcome from all the players and other coaches. The guys come up and give me a hug. I'm thankful for my basketball family. It feels like home. I love to see the guys practicing hard. An hour goes by, and suddenly I'm exhausted. I think I'm going to fall asleep at any moment. I have to go home.

Later that week, I attend an afternoon game and sit in the bleachers behind the bench. I'm able to sit through the entire game, but I leave immediately after to go home and sleep for hours. Every activity leads to extreme exhaustion, to the point where I can't even keep my eyes open. I listen to my body and continue to rest.

Each day that goes by, I can tolerate more and more activity, and I show slight improvement. My strength slowly starts to come back. I don't need to sleep as much anymore. Different nurses come to the house a few times per week to see how my body is recovering from the open-heart surgery. They check my scar and take my vitals. They inspect my Zoll Life Vest to make sure it's working properly. They're happy with what they see. Everything looks the way it should. The nurses urge me to stay patient, listen to my body, and continue to rest.

THIRTY-SIX

Back To Work

A couple of weeks pass and I'm cleared to go back to work, but I'm not allowed to drive yet. I have to rely on people to bring me everywhere and I can't sit on the bench during games until my sternum is healed and my new ICD is placed, but Dr. Link allows me to go into the office. He says I can work for as long as I can tolerate it. So, I go to the office for a few hours each day and sit in the stands during practice. During our home games I manage to sit behind the bench. I love being back with the team. The ushers always reserve the first row of bleachers behind the bench for my family and me. Dr. Link doesn't want me traveling yet, so I watch our road games on my computer. Life is slowly getting back to normal.

On December 14, 2015, we play at Boston University —round three of the rivalry between John and me. I'm still not allowed to sit on the bench for this game or travel with the team, so I drive up to Boston with my parents. I think this is the year we're going to win. Our team is better than their team. This is my chance for revenge.

I walk into the gym and Boston University is warming

up. John comes over to greet me, and I notice he has a patch on his warm up shirt. It says "MP." I look at the rest of his teammates, and they all have the same patch. They're honoring me and everything I've been through. I try to hold back my tears. I can't believe it. It's a wonderful moment for my family and me.

The game starts. My parents sit in their usual seats, behind BU's bench while I sit on the opposite side, behind Quinnipiac's bench. We jump out to a fast start and lead 11-2, but BU battles back and takes a one-point lead with ten minutes remaining in the first half. Both teams have hit their stride and are playing well. We take a four-point lead before John makes a three pointer, cutting our lead to one. We regain control and go into halftime with a 41-36 lead. John has had a solid first half, scoring ten points and making two three-pointers.

At halftime, the Quinnipiac play-by-play and color commentary announcers, Bill Schweizer and Bill Mecca, invite me onto the Quinnipiac radio station to talk about my condition, my brother, and Quinnipiac basketball. I enjoy talking with them, tell them I'm doing well, and especially how badly I need to win this game against John.

In the second half, we lead by as many as eight, but BU keeps the game close. With six minutes left, they finally tie the game up at sixty-three. No one leads by more than three points for the remainder of the game. Every time we get a lead, they tie it up. Then they take a lead, and we strike back to tie the game.

With thirty seconds are on the clock, BU has the ball. The game is tied at sixty-eight. They call timeout. I know John is getting the ball.

BU needs to score just one basket to win the game. We need to get one defensive stop and prevent them from scoring. The horn blows. The timeout is over.

BU inbounds the ball. They start running time off the clock. It ticks down from twenty-nine to twenty, and with fifteen seconds remaining they run their play. John has the ball. He passes it and cuts through the lane. All of a sudden, he runs back toward the ball. His teammate hands it to him on the right side of the floor. He takes two hard dribbles to his left and takes a long, three-point shot over the outstretched arms of our six-foot, nine-inch center. *Swish*. Game over. My brother wins the game again.

The mixed feelings are back, the same ones I felt two years ago when he made a shot to tie the game against us. I want to beat him more than anything, but I know how hard he's worked. I think about John's life for the last three weeks, from getting the phone call from me after his game at Kentucky, to him sitting in the waiting room during my emergency open heart surgery, and then him visiting me every free moment that he had. As disappointed as I am about the game, I can't help but smile. He deserved to make that shot.

THIRTY-SEVEN

Surgery

My surgery is scheduled for January 23, 2015, to get my new ICD placed. Leading up to the surgery, I have a few doctor's appointments to make sure my body is ready. I drive to Tufts and have the PICC line removed from my arm. The nurse tells me to look away and to take a deep breath. As I exhale, she gently pulls the line out. There is no pain, but I feel it sliding down the inside of my arm. When it's removed, I don't want to see what it looks like. I don't want to look, but I can't help myself. I take a quick glance as she disposes the line into the trash. It looks like a long silicone wire. It's hard to believe it was sitting in my arm for the last six weeks. It's such a relief to have it removed.

I also check in with Dr. Link on this visit. He wants to see how I'm feeling and how my scars from the surgery are looking. We don't want to risk infection again. He says everything looks good, with no signs of infection. "You'll be ready for surgery in two weeks," he tells me. In the meantime, he wants to see how my body responds now that I'm off the antibiotics. He has to be sure the infection has completely cleared my system and will not come back.

I get the bloodwork taken in Wallingford, and they send the results to Dr. Link in Boston. The results come back negative. The infection is gone, and I'm ready for surgery.

This time I'm getting a subcutaneous ICD, a new technology. It includes a battery pack on the far-left side of my rib cage, under the skin. It's slightly bigger than my last ICD, but just one wire is attached to the battery. The wire sits directly underneath my skin. The battery will last about eight years.

The advantage of the subcutaneous ICD is the placement of the wire. In my old ICD, the wires directly touched my heart muscle, making a lead extraction a dangerous surgery, which I learned the hard way. The subcutaneous ICD wire is not directly touching my heart muscle. If an infection occurs, and the device needs to be removed, the surgery is significantly less intensive. The location of the subcutaneous ICD also benefits my active lifestyle, because it's tucked away and hidden more. The constant movement of my left arm will not aggravate the device.

Everyone is saying this is a routine surgery, but I've heard that before. I know anything can happen. I'm not taking anything for granted. As usual, Dr. Link will have to test the device after it's placed. I just hope it works. I'm so close to getting my life back. Once this surgery is over, I'll feel closure on this entire ordeal and can get back to living my normal lifestyle.

My parents drive me to the hospital on the morning of the surgery. Everyone feels anxious, especially my family. They have to sit and wait while I'm in the operating room, under anesthesia, with no concept of time. I just go to sleep and I wake up—that's all I know. Last time, things didn't go well, and no one is ready to handle another setback. We *all* desperately need to get this behind us.

I go through the routine. I remove my clothes and put on a hospital gown. The nurses prep me for surgery and wheel me into the cold operating room. Everyone is dressed with masks covering their face. I lie on my back, surrounded by nurses and doctors. Everyone is friendly. I have no idea who is who. I hope this is the last time. 1... 2...3...out.

Meanwhile, my family is in the eerily familiar waiting room. A few hours go by, and Dr. Link enters. It's a gut wrenching feeling—news is coming, but they don't know what kind of news. Thankfully, Dr. Link is visibly happy this time. The surgery is a success.

I wake up groggy from the anesthesia. My mom is sitting next to me. I ask if she's okay, knowing, if I'm okay, she's okay. She relays the message from Dr. Link. He implanted the device, tested it, and it worked perfectly. Relief washes over me, despite my anesthetic haze.

My family stays with me for the remainder of the day. After they leave, as I'm lying in my hospital bed, my immense relief balloons. I feel like I've waged a war these past two months, and it's finally over. I'm hooked up to a morphine pump and still have some anesthesia in me, but a sudden surge of energy rolls through my veins. I can't sleep. I call Conor in California, and we talk for an hour. He finally has to prod me off the phone—I could talk all night.

Dr. Link comes in to check on me. I thank him for everything he's done, not only for me, but also for my family. I know he shares our relief. We've developed a bond over the years, and he empathizes with me. He thanks me for my strength, patience, and fortitude in battling through the recovery. As long as I feel good the next day, he says, I'll be able to go home. No life vest. No backpack. No PICC line. Just me. Soon after he leaves, finally, I slip into a restful sleep.

THIRTY-EIGHT

Back To Life

J ohn has a game the next day. I'm scheduled to be released later that afternoon, so I convince my parents to go to John's game without me. They need to get away from the hospital for a couple of hours. I'll be fine. I can watch the game on my laptop.

I can see the weight has lifted from John's shoulders as I watch him play. This is one of his best games of the season. I'm happy for him. Every basket he makes, I flash my laptop screen a big smile. He finishes the game with twenty-two points. After the game, my parents meet me back to Tufts MC. I feel great. I'm cleared for release. It's time to go home.

I can't wait to get back to work full time at Quinnipiac. And I want to start working out again. but Dr. Link warns me to take things slowly. I have a new piece of metal in my body, he reminds me. It has to settle into place.

On February 5, 2015, we play Monmouth University. It's my first game back on the bench. We play great and win the game 72-52. Three days later, we follow it up with a 91-69 win against Niagara.

We're standing in the locker room after the win and Coach Moore is delivering his post-game talk to the team. I'm so happy to be there. On the wall is a board with the conference standings on it. The numbers are magnetic and, each time we win a conference game, Coach Moore asks the player with the biggest impact on the game to change the number. Tonight, he calls on me to change the number. He hands me the number and I place it on the board. He gives me a moment to talk to the team. I thank them, tell them how much I appreciate their support. Their phone calls and text messages helped me get through my stay in the hospital. Their excitement every time I came to watch practice put a smile on my face. We all put our hands in. I say family on three. "One...two... three...FAMILY!"

That season at Quinnipiac is a roller coaster ride. We have a talented team but can't put together consistent wins. We finish the regular season 15-14 and are ranked sixth in the conference tournament, set to take place in March. We're paired with Marist College, which has some talented players just coming back from injuries. We know it will be a tough game. At the Times Union Center in Albany, NY, after a slow start to the game, we lose 80-74, ending our season.

My biggest physical challenge now is getting back into shape. Before my open-heart surgery, I was happy with my fitness level. I'd had a good workout routine and felt really strong. I understood my limitations with HCM and knew how hard I was able to push my body. But after no exercise for six weeks, two surgeries, and a major infection, I've lost all my gains.

I start to ease back into my workouts, but it's extremely frustrating. I tire quickly. I feel weaker. I'm so far behind and can't keep up. I feel like I'm starting over. This is normal, considering what my body has been through, but I can't accept it. Since my cardiac arrest, workouts have helped my self-image. When I exercise and eat healthy, I feel better. I'm energized and confident, which I've learned is crucial to my overall happiness. I want this feeling back.

I force myself not to compare myself to others or even to the person I was before the open-heart surgery. That person can come back, but it's going to take time, and I have to accept that. There is no reason to compete with anything or anyone besides my current self. I focus on doing this, and it helps immensely.

I start slowly, running very short distances. Every day, I try to run longer and faster. I go to the weight room before work and start lifting very light weights. Each day I try to build back my strength. It feels like progress is happening at a snail's pace, but I'm progressing, so I'm proud of that. I convince myself to keep moving forward. A small progression each day will lead to the ultimate goal of more confidence and happiness. As months go by, I start to notice my gain. Each day, I feel better. Each day, I wake up with more energy. Each day, I'm happier.

THIRTY-NINE

Climbing The Ladder

There's an opportunity for me to get a new job. Scott Burrell, one of the assistants at Quinnipiac, is in the running to be the next head coach at Southern Connecticut State University. I met Scott when I was a freshman and he was a first-year assistant coach at Quinnipiac. Our relationship has grown through my four years as student-manager and three years as the Director of Basketball Operations.

Scott is a legend among UConn basketball fans. He was part of the first Big East Championship team UConn ever had and the first person in sports history to be drafted in the first round of two major professional sports—the NBA and MLB. The Seattle Mariners drafted him as a pitcher in the first round of the Major League Baseball draft following his senior year of high school. He turned down the offer in order to attend college. He was drafted again the following year, in the fifth round. He played some minor league baseball but ultimately loved basketball more. After four years playing basketball at UConn, he was drafted by the Charlotte Hornets as the twentieth overall pick in the 1993 NBA Draft. He played in the NBA for eight seasons, averaging seven points and five rebounds per game for his career. He played on the Charlotte Hornets, New Jersey Nets, Golden State Warriors, and Chicago Bulls. The highlight of his NBA career was playing on the Bulls 1998 NBA Championship team with Michael Jordan. He followed his NBA playing career by playing for five seasons professionally in Japan, China, Spain, and the Philippines, before starting his coaching career at Quinnipiac.

Scott is mentor to me. I look up to him, both figuratively and literally. He's six feet, seven inches tall and boasts the broad frame of a professional athlete. More importantly, he's one of the humblest, kindest human beings I have ever been around. After spending five minutes with him, he makes you feel like family. He has a contagious personality and booming laugh, and he treats everyone with the respect they deserve. He's spoken to me about potentially getting this head coaching job, and he's already offered me his top assistant coach position if he gets it.

Southern CT is a high-level Division 2 program coming off a lot of success. They've reached the NCAA Tournament the previous two years and have a good core of talent coming back. This is a great opportunity for him to be a head coach and for me to move up and be an assistant. I'm ready to make the jump.

Scott's interview process is long. It drags out for weeks. The school has strict hiring policies in place, and they must be followed. Rumors are spreading that Scott is getting the job, but nothing becomes official for weeks.

Scott is named the head coach at Southern CT State University on July 13, 2015. I meet with Coach Moore before leaving to accept Scott's offer, and he agrees this is the next step in my career. We have a mutual respect for each other. Coach Moore knows how special Quinnipiac is to me. I've spent seven long years of my life working for the team and have experienced a lot of ups and downs with the program. Quinnipiac University basketball has been, and always will be, a true family. The relationships created will last forever. I was there when Coach Moore started his first season, and it's bittersweet leaving him, but I have to take this step forward. We shake hands knowing this isn't the end of our relationship. I'll be back for practices and games. I promise to do whatever he needs while he searches for my replacement.

Scott and I have our work cut out for us at SCSU. School starts in six weeks, and we need to recruit four new players in the two weeks left in the recruiting period. We have to find and evaluate our prospects quickly. We head out on the recruiting trail and contact our coaching network to find kids still looking for schools to attend in the fall. We travel up and down the Northeast, watching hundreds of AAU basketball games. We find a handful of kids we want to come play for us and we do research on them, looking at their grades and talking to their high school and AAU coaches. We want to make sure they're good people we want representing our program.

August is spent on campus giving tours to the potential recruits and selling them on our school. We invite our returning players to come for the visit, so the recruits can get to know their possible future teammates. Four players commit. They apply and are admitted to school. We have our roster set for the upcoming season.

FORTY

Assistant Coach

We start our Fall workouts on September 1, 2015. We have a very talented team at Southern CT, and the opposing coaches vote us to finish first in a pre-season poll. We have two of the best players in the country as our leading scorers and a great group of role players surrounding them.

Our season gets off to a hot start. We're 5-0 before taking our first loss to our cross-town rivals, University of New Haven. It's a bad loss, but an eye opener for our players. We know now not to underestimate anyone. We finish the regular season as conference champions, with an overall record of 22-6. Our conference record is 17-3.

John is in his senior year of college and I visit him as much as I can. This is the last year I can watch him play at this level. He's considering attempting a professional career overseas, but that's unknown. He finishes his career in remarkable fashion, scoring 1,289 points, finishing second in school history for 3-pointers made with 287, setting the school record for most 3-pointers made in one season at 95, setting the school record for most games played over the course of a career, and setting the record for best assist-to-turnover ratio. I'm so proud of him.

We enter the conference tournament that year with hopes to win a championship, but it won't be easy. The league is very competitive. In our opening round game against Southern New Hampshire we jump out to an eighteen-point lead early in the second half. Everything is going right for us, but then the tide turns as Southern New Hampshire slowly starts chipping away at the lead. We're up by just one point with thirty seconds remaining and have to stop them from scoring one more time to win the game. We get a steal, and one of our players drives the ball down the court for an uncontested dunk. We start to celebrate with five seconds remaining on the clock. There is no way we can lose. Then, one of their players makes one of the best plays I've ever seen. He grabs the ball out of the net and immediately throws it down the court to one of his teammates, their best shooter, who has his head down thinking his team has lost.

The pass is perfect. He picks his head up, catches the pass, and takes a shot at the buzzer. Nothing but net. Tie game. Overtime. With the dramatic change in momentum, SNH goes on to win in overtime.

It's the most crushing loss I've ever been a part of as a coach, but the season overall has been successful. I love working with Scott and being around the students. It seems to be a good fit, but I start to think about my life and what I really want my future to look like. I have put a lot of time into coaching, but I'm unsure if this is my true passion.

FORTY-ONE

In A Heartbeat

After my cardiac arrest, my family, friends, and I dreamed of starting our own non-profit organization. In the years since I collapsed, we talked about it often but never took any steps toward making it a reality. I promised myself that, after my open-heart surgery, I'd make this dream come true. I needed to use my life experiences to help others and save more lives.

First, we need a dynamic name for our organization. My mom always talks about how her life changed "in a heartbeat" when she received the phone call from my dad on the day of my cardiac arrest. The perfect name: In A Heartbeat.

Incorporating as a nonprofit is a long and arduous task. The paperwork has to be filed perfectly, so we want to hire lawyers to ensure the quality of the filing process. But lawyers are expensive, and we haven't raised any money yet, so we launch a campaign via Facebook using a company that drop ships t-shirts. We sell the shirts for twenty dollars. The company gets a portion and we get a portion to cover the startup costs of our organization. The campaign is a huge hit. We raise close to $5,000 in t-shirt sales.

We immediately hire a group of nonprofit lawyers to file paperwork to the IRS. It takes a couple of meetings, but we gather information, organize paperwork, then file and wait for a response. We're officially recognized as a 501 (c) 3 corporation on October 2, 2015. Our mission is to prevent death from sudden cardiac arrest and Hypertrophic Cardiomyopathy.

We create four main programs to fulfill our mission. First is our *AED Donation Program*. We donate AEDs to schools, businesses, and other organizations in need. We also provide CPR/AED Training and assist with setting up emergency action plans. With our *Hypertrophic Cardiomyopathy Research Funding Program*, we donate money to various research projects throughout the country dedicated to furthering the overall knowledge and treatment of Hypertrophic Cardiomyopathy. Our *Patient Support Program* provides support to heart disease patients, cardiac arrest survivors, patients with an implanted defibrillator, and their families. Finally, our *Cardiac Screening Program* provides free ECGs to children, teens, and young adults.

This is just a part time hobby for me. I'm still an assistant coach at Southern CT. But any time I'm not coaching, I'm trying to help In A Heartbeat grow. Eventually, news of our work starts to spread throughout our local community. People send in donations, and we donate our first AED to Manchester Knights Youth Sports and Cheerleading Program on May 3, 2016. On September 27 of that year we host our first golf tournament fundraiser, and on October 31, we donate six thousand dollars to Tufts Medical Center and the Hypertrophic Cardiomyopathy Center, a place I'm very familiar with.

As the days go on, my life passion starts to shift.

Coaching takes up so much of my time. It used to be all that mattered to me, but now I want to give more time to In A Heartbeat. We're in the middle of another successful season at Southern CT, and I spend all day in the office and at practice. I spend my nights calling recruits and creating scouting reports for our opponents. Oftentimes, when I'm done working, I'm too tired to put any effort into In A Heartbeat. The organization should be growing faster. We're doing great work but we can always impact more people.

I tell myself my calling is coaching. I've spent the last nine years building an impressive resumé--Student Manager at Quinnipiac, Assistant Coach at UMass Lowell, Director of Basketball Operations at Quinnipiac, and Assistant Coach at Southern CT State University. I'm still relatively young to be an assistant coach, and I'm in a position to possibly become a head coach at the collegiate level someday. I can't stop coaching in college now—it doesn't make sense. This is difficult to come to terms with. It's hard for me to understand that it's okay and normal for my passion in life to change. Just because it doesn't make sense for me to stop coaching doesn't mean I should continue to do something I don't truly love to do anymore.

As In A Heartbeat grows, I start to speak publicly more and more. I learn about the speaking industry and believe there is a place for me. I can help people by sharing my story and my experiences in life.

I want to be out there sharing my story more. I want to inspire others. At night, after I finish my coaching duties, I study how to become a professional motivational speaker. I read books and watch videos. I take online classes. Through a mutual friend from Tufts, I connect with a very successful speaker and author, Mark Leblanc, who agrees to have a virtual meeting with me. He gives me hope that I have a future in the speaking industry. He tells me to start by getting in front of local athletic directors in Connecticut. Given my athletic and coaching career, this is a good place to start. He also helps me develop my speech. He knows my story is powerful, but people aren't going to hire me to just tell my story. There are a lot of great stories out there. They're going to hire me to help improve production by their employees, their students, or their athletes. It's necessary to develop a speech that includes my story, but more importantly, what I've learned along the way, and how it will benefit the audience. The speech is not about *me*. It's about the *audience*. This meeting with Mark inspires me, and I immediately get to work.

We finish the 2016-17 season strong with an overall record of 18-13 and a conference record of 13-7. Our leading scorer is nominated to the All-Conference Team. We're invited to play in the Division Two NCAA Tournament. But I feel relieved when the season ends after a second-round loss in the NCAA Tournament—I know I'll have more time to focus on In A Heartbeat and my speaking career.

I reach out to the president of the Connecticut Association of Athletic Directors and tell him I want to be the keynote speaker at their spring conference. He agrees to give me a chance. Every athletic director in the state will be there. If I can nail my talk in front of them, I'll be invited to speak at their schools. My first keynote speech is scheduled on March 24, 2017. It will be a sixty minute speech titled "Attack Your Dreams."

Prior to the speech, Scott and I fly to Chicago to go recruiting. There's a Junior College tournament we want to watch. As I drive to Bradley International Airport to meet Scott, my focus is on my upcoming talk. I don't think about the trip. I can't wait to get back. I practice my speech over and over again. It has to be perfect. After spending three days in Chicago watching games, I fly home. I have one more day to prepare, so I practice my speech all day. I walk around my neighborhood reciting it aloud. I practice in the mirror, watching my movements and my mannerisms. I feel like I'm watching film of an opponent as I critique myself.

I wake up early on the morning of the talk, which is scheduled for 8:30 a.m. I want to practice once more before I leave, so I arrive at the conference early. The room is big and filled with a lot of people. They offer me breakfast, but I'm not hungry. My stomach is nervous. It's the same feeling I get before I coach a game. I sit in the front row for my introduction. I feel ready to go. My adrenaline is flowing through my body. When my name is called, I stand up and take the microphone. All eyes are on me. It's showtime.

I tell my story, which I've done countless times before. It's easy. I can tell nobody in the audience can believe all I've been through medically. I look too young. After my own story, I transition to the lessons I've learned. I've learned a lot in my life, and I know the audience can apply my life lessons to their own personal life. I make a joke about how I use the fact that I literally have a big heart as a pick-up line when out at a bar with my friends. Everyone laughs. I talk about stepping out of your comfort zone, making an impact, working hard, being nice, and fighting the feeling of regret. I have a notecard in my pocket in case I forget something, but I don't. I spent too much time practicing to forget any of the points I want to make. After fifty-five minutes, I wrap it up. When I say, "Thank-you," the audience stands and applauds. A standing ovation. Just what I needed. I listen to them clap and feel proud of myself, but the only thing that comes to mind is: When can I do this again?

I'm now sure it's time for me to make a change. The feelings of not being excited to go into work have turned into feelings of anxiety. My body is telling me the time to shift paths has come. I need to step away from college coaching. I think about what will happen if I quit. I earn a nice salary. That will be gone. How will I pay my bills? I'm on track to be a head coach someday. If I quit, that opportunity will disappear. I work at a great university with a close friend. What if I ruin my relationship with him? Maybe it doesn't make sense to quit. Maybe I should stick it out.

I also think about my life passions. What am I most excited to do every single day? Going to work at Southern CT does not excite me like In A Heartbeat does. It does not give me a burning passion like speaking does. I know that if I don't give this new passion a chance while I'm still young, I'll regret it for the rest of my life. I almost died twice in my life. I understand how valuable each and every day is. I understand true happiness and what I need to do to find it.

The decision is made. If it doesn't work, I can always say I tried.

The hardest part of this decision is talking to Scott. I feel like I'm letting him down. I don't want him to be mad at me for leaving the program. I don't want to ruin a relationship with a great friend. I know I have to do it, and the longer I wait, the harder it will be to have the conversation.

In April, we're both in the office. I have a huge pit in my stomach. I know today is the day. We have post-season meetings scheduled with our players. I'll talk to Scott after the meetings. The meetings end. He stands up to go home for the day, and I tell him I need to talk to him about something. He sits back down and listens.

"I have to talk to you about something," I say to him. "This is a hard conversation for me to have. I don't want to ruin our friendship."

Scott replies, "What's going on? Is everything ok?"

I start to get emotional and say, "I care about you and this program but I have to step away to focus on In A Heartbeat and my speaking career. I believe running this nonprofit and speaking are my true passions in life."

Scott looks at me and smiles saying, "You have to do what makes you happy. I can not be mad at you for doing what makes you truly happy."

We stand up and embrace with a hug. I thank him for everything he has done to mentor and support me. Another sign of the type of person and the type of friend Scott is. I tell him I appreciate his support and promise to stay with him until he hires someone else.

The conversation ends, and I feel better. I'm ready to take on the next journey of my life. I'm ready to attack my dream. I'm ready to SAVE LIVES.

FORTY-TWO

The Next Chapter

As I finish writing this book, I have begun my next chapter in life. I have seen my dreams and goals change several times in my thirty-plus years of life, from becoming a college basketball player to being a physical therapist, from becoming a college basketball coach to starting my own non-profit foundation, from full-time professional speaking, to writing a book.

Some of my dreams I have achieved, and some I hope to achieve someday. And though there is one dream I'll never achieve—playing basketball in college—in a way, I have achieved this dream tenfold. Every game I've coached, I put myself in the shoes of every player on the court. I celebrated their wins, ached for their losses, and took tremendous pride in helping to shape their collegiate athletic careers.

My inability to play college basketball turned out to be the root of every subsequent dream—the catalyst to each achievement I've worked so hard for. Sometimes, on the flip side of our greatest losses, we find opportunity to create our greatest wins.

Epilogue

I n A Heartbeat is diligently working to prevent death from sudden cardiac arrest and Hypertrophic Cardiomyopathy. At the time this book was published we have donated 177 Automated External Defibrillators to different schools, businesses, families, and organizations in need. Although we often donate in Connecticut, we have also donated AEDs throughout the United States. We have also donated $35,000 to help fund various Hypertrophic Cardiomyopathy research projects and have started a support group for heart disease patients, cardiac arrest survivors, patients with an implanted defibrillator, and their families. We have launched our Cardiac Screening Program and offer free ECGs to children, teens, and young adults. Our hope is to continue to grow, impact more people, and help SAVE LIVES!

My speaking career has grown tremendously as well. My speaking gig at the CAAD Conference, in particular, opened many doors for me. I've been lucky enough to speak at high schools, universities, and corporate businesses. I've spoken in Connecticut, New York, Massachusetts, Pennsylvania, Florida, Illinois, Louisiana, Tennessee, and Washington. I hope to continue to build my speaking career nationally and speak at both the university and coprorate levels. I truly believe my story and what I've learned from my experiences can positively impact audiences of all ages.

I'm living a very normal life with HCM. I'm confident with my ICD and feel safe with it. I've gotten myself into good physical shape and am comfortable with my workout routine and eating habits. I go to the gym and do a healthy mix of running, biking, light weight-lifting, yoga, and core power. I still take Nadolol two times per day to control my heart rate, my blood pressure, and most importantly to help prevent ventricular fibrillation and another sudden cardiac arrest. I get my ICD interrogated three or four times per year. Soon, I'll have surgery to get my battery replaced in my ICD. With the new ICD I'll only need to get the device interrogated once per year at the doctor's office because of a system that sends updates virtually so the hospital can monitor me from home. Pretty amazing. Dr. Heller, a pediatric cardiologist, agreed to see me as a patient through college. She is still involved with the work we do with In A Heartbeat. Now, I only meet with Dr. Maron once a year to check in. Currently, nothing has changed. The thickness of my heart has stayed consistent, and I have not developed any other symptoms. I'm lucky that my life is very normal.

I'm the President and Founder of In A Heartbeat. On April 7, 2018, I was named the Head Basketball Coach at Fairfield College Preparatory School, a Jesuit high school in Fairfield, CT. It's a part time job and allows me to focus my time on all three of my passions: In A Heartbeat, speaking, and coaching. My dad is one of my assistant coaches, making the job even more special. I also work for

Defibtech, a CT based AED manufacturing company in the role of Manager of Community Relations. I truly am lucky to work in all different aspects of the Automated External Defibrillator industry.

John graduated from Boston University with a degree in International Relations in 2016. He got a job doing inside sales with a cybersecurity company in Waltham, MA called Carbon Black. It was a great job for a new graduate, but he didn't love it. At the end of the year, he quit and went back to be the Video Coordinator at Boston University for the Men's Basketball Team and to get his Masters Degree in Project Management. After one year in that role, he was promoted to Director of Basketball Operations. Since then, he decided to step away from coaching and currently works as a Customer Success Manager at Zappi, an automated market research platform. He is still in the gray area in terms of developing HCM. Doctors think he would have shown signs of the disease by this point in his life, but there is no way to be sure since the genetic testing results still show a genetic variant of uncertain significance. He follows up with Dr. Maron yearly and receives an electrocardiogram and echocardiogram at his visits.

My mom and dad ended up separating but our family still spends time together, which is really special for all of us. My dad is still working as a conductor for Metro North, and my mom has held multiple roles in the Wallingford School System, including Department Head for Special Education, Director of the Integrated Pre-School, and of course, teaching.

Conor and I are still best friends. I go out to Los Angeles at least once a year, and he comes home for the holidays and for some time in the summer. He still plays in various men's basketball leagues in LA every night of the week and calls me every time he has a good game. His competitive drive has never gone away. He worked for BNY Wealth Management for about six years before going back to school full time to get his Masters of Business Administration at the University of Southern California. After graduation he accepted a job working as an Associate in the Investment Banking Division for Credit Suisse.

Bob and I remain close. Our families get together every year on the anniversary of my sudden cardiac arrest. He is a breast cancer survivor and I had the opportunity to take him for chemotherapy and tried to be there for him like he was for me on August 24, 2006. Although he calls himself a regular guy, he still looks like Superman to me.

Acknowledgments

As with everything else in my life, this memoir would not have been possible without the love and support of many people. I would not be the person I am today without the loving support of my mother, my father, and my brother, John. On page 1, I wrote, "It is always harder on the family than it is on the patient." That couldn't be more true. I don't remember going into sudden cardiac arrest. I don't remember suffering through open-heart surgery. But they do. They recall it too clearly…like it was yesterday. They can still feel the agony of not knowing if I would live or die. Reliving these moments as I gathered information for this memoir brought my family back to a dark place—a place they fight every day not to return to. I am forever grateful to them for revisiting this pain to allow me to share my story with you.

Though I refer to Conor throughout the book as my best friend, at this point, he is really my brother. We were beside each other the moment I collapsed in cardiac arrest and have remained present for each other ever since. I know now it isn't common to stay so close to your childhood best friend. I couldn't be more grateful to be one of the lucky few.

Quite literally, I would not be here today if not for Bob Huebner. In addition to physically saving my life, Bob has supported my every endeavor since my cardiac arrest. He calls me his third son…and I wear that moniker like a badge of honor.

There is no way I would have been able to complete this book without the help of a long line of people. Dr. Felice Heller, Dr. Ramesh Iyer, Dr. Martin Maron, Dr. Mark Link, and Noreen Dolan, NP-C, not only kept me alive at critical moments of my life, they helped me get my life back. We stay in touch and whenever I reach out, they invariably greet me with excitement and energy. While juggling time with family, treating patients, and performing surgery, they each took the time to review this memoir for medical accuracy—a crucial detail to appropriately support heart disease patients navigating their own personal journeys.

To the rest of my friends and family: I could write an entire *second* book about the impact you have had on my life. If I didn't write in depth about you in this memoir, please know how much I appreciate you!

I can't adequately express how deeply grateful I am to everyone who visited me in the hospital—your endless stream of drop-ins, calls, cards, and prayers lifted me and my family more than words can express. Thank you for your support and for helping me get through some of the most challenging weeks of my life.

There were many times over the last couple of years when I felt like I could not finish this memoir. Thank you to my two editors, Natasha Blanchard and Chris Belden. Without your skill, expertise, support, and motivation, this memoir might still be just an in-progress file on my computer.

Thank you to the In A Heartbeat Board of Directors who have worked diligently to grow our tiny nonprofit into an organization with tremendous impact. Your dedicated support of our mission has helped us save so many lives, and I am so grateful.

Finally, thank *you* for taking the time to read my story. While writing this memoir, one thought stayed in my mind. This isn't about me—it isn't about my story. This is about *you*, reading these words, and how *you* can cull lessons I learned the hard way and hopefully have a positive impact on your own life somehow. Thank you for giving me the incredible opportunity to do that!

Contact Mike Papale

In A Heartbeat

If In A Heartbeat can support you, a family member, a friend, or an organization you are involved with please do not hesitate to reach out to us. If you wish to donate to our life saving mission, you can do by visiting our web site. Our web site is inaheartbeat.org and you can contact Mike directly via email at mike@inaheartbeat.org.

Hire Mike To Speak

If you are interested in hiring Mike to speak at your next event, please visit his personal web site at michaelpapale.com. You can also send him an email directly at mike@michaelpapale.com.

A Big Heart Podcast

Mike is the host of A Big Heart, a podcast about living with heart disease. This podcast dissects the physical and emotional obstacles that a patient endures while living with heart disease. The goal is to help heart disease patients of all ages live a long and normal life! The podcast is available Apple Podcasts, Spotify, and all other streaming platforms.

Social Media

Facebook.com/mike.papale.1
Twitter: @Mike_Papale
Instagram: @mikepapale

CPSIA information can be obtained
at www.ICGtesting.com
Printed in the USA
LVHW032343011221
704984LV00008B/1358